FASTING

A GUIDE TO HEALTH AND WELLNESS

BRYAN MCASKILL

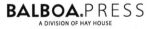
BALBOA.PRESS
A DIVISION OF HAY HOUSE

Balboa Press books may be ordered through booksellers or by contacting:

Balboa Press
A Division of Hay House
1663 Liberty Drive
Bloomington, IN 47403
www.balboapress.com
844-682-1282

Print information available on the last page.

ISBN: 978-1-9822-5679-1 (sc)
ISBN: 978-1-9822-5680-7 (e)

Balboa Press rev. date: 10/27/2020

CONTENTS

Chapter 1   What Is Fasting? 1

Chapter 2   Is Fasting For You? 9

Chapter 3   Most Common Fasting Methods 15

Chapter 4   Preparing To Fast 19

Chapter 5   How Long To Fast 25

Chapter 6   Using Sleep To Your Advantage 29

Chapter 7   Should I Exercise While Fasting? 35

Chapter 8   Sample Fasting Routines vs Cleansing
            and Detoxing 39

Chapter 9   Cleanses and Detoxes 77

Chapter 10 Breathe 117

Chapter 11 Why Your Powers Increase When
            Fasting 137

Chapter 12 Final Thoughts 141

CHAPTER 1

What Is Fasting?

Fasting, "is an abstinence from food, or a limiting of one's food, especially when voluntary and/or as a religious observance." Fasting will not harm you or damage your body when facilitated correctly. Many people undertake extended fasts to cleanse their system and cure their diseases. Your body is a container for the soul. It must be kept clean and pure so that it can heal itself when given the right conditions. Many strongholds are broken while fasting, mental clarity improves, addictions are broken, manifestation is quicker, natural beauty is restored, unwanted soul ties are cut loose, intuition is sharper, and a stronger connection to the Higher Self is achieved.

Fasting has existed since the beginning of life on Earth. An ill or injured animal's first instinct is to abstain from

1

solid food until it is again healthy. They instinctively know that the healing process will be much faster and more effective when it abstains from solid food that will burden its digestive tract. This instinct has always existed within the animal kingdom. The human body also has this same instinct, for it is common for most people to stop eating when illness strikes. Fasting has been both used as a religious ritual (connection) and for preventing and curing diseases. Fasting purifies the body of the Earth's wide variety of natural and unnatural pollutants thereby improving bodily health and function.

Fasting improves the body's capacity and ability to better utilize the food eaten after a fast.

When the body gets no rest from processing food day after day, the digestive and cleansing systems are often subject to an interrupted workload and can lead to plaque which prevents nutritional absorption. The body is often unable to rid itself of all these stored toxins, waste products, body acids, excess proteins, and fat deposits. If this condition continues long enough, it can lead to innumerable diseases.

Fasting can and should be the foundation of any diet or lifestyle. It is necessary to give the digestive system a rest, and more importantly to clean the body. Fasting will free up energy you typically spend digesting foods throughout the day. Rather than digesting things during the day, the body shifts it's focus on renewing and repairing itself. How much sense does it make to have a closet full of clutter, but continue to buy new things you try to fit in there? You would want to first get rid of anything you do not need so you understand what you already have and be able to decide what you may need. The body works the same way. Fasting gives the organs a much needed and much deserved rest and help the body heal quicker.

During a fast, many biochemical processes will take place in the body, resulting in many reactions outside the body as well. These metabolic processes will take place whether you supply the body with food or not. When fasting, the body will start releasing low-grade energy stored as fat, which will rapidly decrease body fat levels. This fat is the bad fat (white fat), not the healthy fat (brown fat) that is crucial to our brain, organ, and muscle development.

Fasting can prevent, improve, and also work to cure many conditions such as circulatory problems, diabetes, intestinal problems, tumors and cancer cells, correct respiratory conditions, skin problems and much more; especially when accompanied with a whole food, plant-based lifestyle.

Fasting is a practice that has had a recent rise in popularity in the last few years, even though it dates back for centuries, and plays a central role in many cultures and religions. The late healer Dr. Sebi (Alfredo Bowman) himself was a huge advocate of fasting, and he would do it frequently to maximize the healing and cleansing benefits from his cell food compounds.

Dr. Sebi use to accompany his fasts with agua de tamarindo (tamarind water) when he was not ingesting solid foods. He also consumed certain products like his Green Food and Bromide Plus products to nourish his cells in his body. Green Food amplifies the blood-purifying and cleansing effects of fasting, while also strengthening and improving the respiratory, digestive, immune, and nervous system; Bromide Plus is a great energizer and revitalizer, and it has all the necessary nutrients and minerals, so they are both great products to complement and sustain the body during a fast. The concept of removing what is not needed, while concurrently feeding your cells to achieve optimum health and longevity is essentially the core concept of fasting. I strongly recommend that you start by following the *Dr. Sebi Nutritional Guide* and let your body adapt slowly to it.

Start off by skipping one meal a day until you build up to a full day (if you can) and proceed from there when you're ready to plan for a fast after you have built up your tolerance. Always make sure to break a fast during the window of time that you can eat. When you fast, digestion and other metabolic functions are put on hold. All energy goes towards healing and cleansing your body, so it is vital to break the fast with the proper foods. Soups, smoothies, and juices. Making these items based on Dr. Sebi's Nutritional Guide are ideal since they are nutrient-dense and easy to digest.

Most Common Benefits Of Fasting

Fasting has helped many people reach their health goals and improve their overall lifestyle. Here are five of the most common benefits that people experience while fasting:

1) Fasting Promotes Blood-Sugar Control. By decreasing insulin resistance, which means your body is more effective at transporting glucose from your bloodstream to your cells, fasting improves blood-sugar control. This benefit is more clearly found in short-term intermittent fasting; for example, abstaining from food for 16 hours a day, and eating within an eight-hour window. Since the blood always tries to keep its level of protein constant, it will keep these levels up by breaking down inferior tissues of diseases, damaged, aged, or dead cells, abnormal growth tissues, tumors, and other undesirable tissues.

2) Fasting Fights Inflammation. Inflammation is a side effect of consuming too many acidic-forming foods, toxins, or by being around a toxic environment. Inflammation is also involved in the development

of chronic conditions, such as heart disease, cancer, multiple sclerosis, and rheumatoid arthritis. By fasting for close to twelve hours a day, it is possible to reduce inflammation without medications and without side effects, which helps to naturally aid in treating the diseases mentioned above. This does not have to be a daily thing or carried out forever. But, it should be considered more of a norm for those with any of these conditions.

3) Fasting Enhances Heart Health. Heart disease is one of the leading causes of death around the world. By making lifestyle changes, such as following Dr. Sebi's Nutritional Guide, and incorporating fasting into your daily routine, it is possible to decrease high blood pressure, triglycerides, and cholesterol, all of which can lead to heart disease.

4) Fasting Boosts Brain Function. Fasting does good things for the brain, and this is evident by all the beneficial neuro-chemical changes that happen in the brain when we fast. Fasting improves cognitive function, increases neurotrophic factors and stress resistance, and works to reduce inflammation. You can boost the brain benefits of fasting by consuming natural healing herbs while you fast. Herbs such as, Burdock Root, Sarsaparilla, Guaco, Tumba Vaquero, Santa Maria, Blue Vervain, Valerian Root, among others, helps stimulate the brain and helps in the treatment of diseases related to the central nervous

system, such as depression, anxiety, irritability, and insomnia.

5) Fasting Can Delay Aging and Increase Longevity. Fasting regularly has been proven to delay aging and increase longevity to those who practice it along with other healthy lifestyle choices. The body's production of human growth hormones and metabolism increases after an extended fast and stays higher than normal for a longer period of time. This stimulates greater muscle growth, keeps us younger and creates higher fat metabolism, which is the burning and removal of excess fat and toxic cells.

6) Stimulates Autophagy. The process of "Autophagy" was brought to mainstream when Biologist, Yoshinori Oshumi was awarded the Nobel prize for its discovery in 2016. Autophagy literally means "to eat oneself". This is the body's mechanism of getting rid of all the broken down, old cell machinery when there is no longer enough energy to sustain it. During this process, the body breaks down unhealthy fat, cysts, and toxins. Fasting is more beneficial than just stimulating autophagy for the fact that fasting can be extended and performed in a variety of ways. By stimulating autophagy, we are clearing out the old proteins and cellular parts. During this same time, fasting also stimulates growth hormones, which tell our body to start producing some new cells for the body. Instead of taking in nutrients, cells undergoing

autophagy can recycle the damaged parts they have, remove toxic material, and repair themselves. Autophagy encourages growth of new brain cells and protects the nervous system and nerve cells.

Fasting can be, and is a very enjoyable experience for those who take it upon themselves to embark upon this adventure. Fasting is a process that involves building up your tolerance, while staying dedicated and mindful to your intentions during this time period. You will want to remain prepared, and not be too concerned with breaking your fast unless it is needed. Like anything else in life, the most important part is to simply get started.

CHAPTER 2

Is Fasting For You?

Outside of a dry fast, all types of fasting allow drinking water or other liquids, like herbal tea, juices, and smoothies. Whatever type of fast you decide to do, you might experience some symptoms that are listed below which are better to know of in advance so you can prepare mentally and physically for them.

1) Hunger. As you start a fast and skip your first regular time that you eat, it is likely that you will experience hunger. Your digestive system and organs are used to working on a specific schedule you have developed over time which will make you feel your body adjusting and can feel uneasy or uncomfortable. This may initially lead to mood swings, decreased energy levels, and irritability, among other symptoms. All these symptoms are

completely normal, as your body is beginning to experience a process known as "Gluconeogenesis". During Gluconeogenesis, your liver switches its role from converting sugar to now converting non-carbohydrate materials like lactate, amino acids, and fats into glucose for energy. At this stage, you might feel drained as your basal metabolic rate, heart rate, and blood pressure lowers, but stick to it as you will adjust to this stage. Think of your body beginning to power down its normal way of functioning and creating a new energy source.

2) Less Hunger And More Energy. This stage comes once your body has adapted to gluconeogenesis and begins a process known as "ketosis". Ketosis happens when your body starts to burn stored fat as its primary power source, and your normal energy levels return. Once the ketosis process begins, a lot of the benefits of fasting start to happen as well like weight loss and detoxification. Fat stores are used to storing toxic metals and other toxins, so during the Ketosis process, the body can focus on expelling these from your body. I am not advocating a Ketogenic diet or lifestyle as most of those foods used or that type of diet are acidic and mucus forming which will become detrimental to your health. I am however, promoting the natural Ketosis process by fasting in addition to following the foods from the Nutritional Guide which consist of Alkaline foods that are natural and original to this planet.

3) Fatigue, Diarrhea, Congestion, Skin Breakouts. The detoxification process from fasting can be rough at times on your body, especially if this is new to you. Your body is expelling toxins accumulated in your fat stores, and delivering them into your bloodstream, impacting on your well-being. The more regularly you fast and eat to feed your cells, the blood will become cleaner; there are also many herbs you can incorporate into your lifestyle that can clean the blood which we will go over later. Your body is adapting to a new normal in which you may feel fatigue, congestion, and/or diarrhea. This is a good thing as you will become more in tune with what your body needs and learn to adapt to these changes. It should be noted that, if you are new to fasting, you will not be fasting for an extended period of time so you may not end up noticing these responses immediately. The detoxification process triggers the worst symptoms of a fast: fatigue, diarrhea, congestion, skin breakouts, mood swings, nausea, irritability, stuffy nose, etc. This "healing crisis" varies from person to person, depending on different factors like how poor your eating habits were before the fast, but it usually lasts for up to three days. It will be best for your overall health to weather this storm to build up your tolerance for what is next in your process.

Depending on the type of fast you are doing, key lime juice and herbal teas may help flush out toxins and provide nutrients and antioxidants, relieving the symptoms. This stage can be tough, but you will get through this!

4) Emotional Detox. Repressed emotions can also surface when you are going through a fast. Unpleasant feelings might appear since you are putting your body through a great deal of stress. Do not be surprised if you have certain memories or feelings like anxiety, depression, sadness, frustration, and resentment come up during your fast. Keep in mind that as these emotions and feelings arise, you are being granted the opportunity to relieve yourself in-the-moment of this burden as you process what thoughts may come to the surface. You cannot heal what you do not bring into your awareness. Remind yourself to be thankful and grateful to your body for bringing these items to the surface for you to work on bettering yourself during this healing process. You can relieve these symptoms by upping up your self-care routine also. Journaling, massages, music, and meditation may become more present in your life as daily routines to adopt during this time which may also be helpful. Be extra kind to yourself, and stay strong!

5) Mental Clarity. When your body is not busy trying to digest things, it is able to relax physically as well as mentally. The brain's "plasticity" increases which helps the brain respond quicker to new information. This improves your memory, learning ability, and

mood. You may find yourself thinking more existentially and being able to shift your focus more on the here and now. Worrying, having concerns, and stress begin to diminish more frequently without as much effort.

6) Weight Loss. Fasting makes you more efficient in the process of burning bad fat for energy. Your appetite can go through a healthy change during this time. Your body can do more with less and work to hold onto what it needs and reject what is does not. This makes it easier to stick to an eating plan, and ultimately, helps you lose or maintain a healthy weight.

7) More Energy. After your body adjusts to the complicated processes of gluconeogenesis and ketosis, you will have a ton of sustainable energy from your body's fat stores. You might have felt depleted and fatigued in earlier stages, but once you adjust, you will have more energy that will help continue to push you forward in your transition towards a healthier lifestyle.

8) Clear Complexion and Brighter Skin. Fasting helps to improve blood circulation and promotes healing, which will result in brighter skin and fewer acne-scars. If the blood contains toxins, skin blemishes and acne will remain. When the blood is clean, the skin will remain clean and stay clear; along with remaining hydrated of course.

9) Confidence. As you progress through your fast, you will work through difficulties, remain consistent, and notice every day positive changes you are responsible for creating. You will be proud of yourself for staying consistent and working through this experience. Knowing that you have worked through a fast, you will feel more confident as you try your next one.

10) Healing. This is the most important benefit of fasting. Fasting not only removes toxins and obstructions, it helps the body to heal itself. This is the ultimate goal of a fast. Once you have freed all toxins from your body and you have given your digestive system a very much needed rest, your body can begin to heal from the inside out. In a fasting state, the body will scour for dead cells, damaged tissues, fatty deposits, tumors, all of which are burned for fuel or expelled as waste. Fasting allows a deep, physiological rest of the digestive organs, and the energy saved goes into self-healing and self-repairing.

CHAPTER 3

Most Common Fasting Methods

INTERMITTENT FASTING

Offers alternative regimens for fasting, such as alternate day fasting, one meal per day, or an extended period of time each day where one can fast. As the name implies, it is alternating between periods of eating normally and periods of fasting. These "periods" are open to user definition. Intermittent Fasting is most referred to as the "16:8" method as you fast for 16-hours daily, while leaving the remaining 8-hours to consume foods and only drink water outside of those 8 hours. 16:8 is the goal when doing Intermittent Fasting however, many people adjust the hours to fit in better with their schedule such as 14:10, 12:12, or even 20:4 at times. This fasting method also allows for a complete 24-hour fast, a 36-hour fast, or a schedule which involves skipping an entire meal during a certain day of the week, and at times can lead to a person eating every other day (also known as "Alternate Day Fasting"). The main difference Intermittent Fasting has opposed to other fasting methods is, that other fasting methods will fully restrain from solid foods, while Intermittent Fasting allows for solid foods to be consumed, but only during a specific section of each day within each 24-hour time period.

PARTIAL FASTING

Also sometimes called "selective fasting", partial fasting includes some solid food anywhere from a little to a lot of solid food. It is not the amount of food, but the exclusion or limitation of certain foods that makes it a partial fast. During this fast, you are fasting from specific items to help promote dietary changes as you make a transition to a healthier lifestyle. This fasting method is essentially Intermittent Fasting, just without a regular schedule attached to it.

JUICE FASTING

Is extremely popular and offers a modicum of nutritional support in a pure and natural form. Almost any fruit or vegetable from the Dr. Sebi Nutritional

Guide can be juiced with the powerful juicers on the market. A juice fast is helpful for those who wish to satisfy current taste buds to make fasting a bit easier and make sure to load up on vital nutrients and minerals while staying hydrated.

LIQUID FASTING

As the name implies, this is fasting on liquids only. Typically consists of a mix of select herbal teas or bitters, together with minerals and natural spring water. This form of fasting allows for smoothies, juices, and herbal teas in which you can express your creativity and test out different combinations of flavors.

WATER FASTING

Natural spring water fasting is the simplest and perhaps the oldest form of liquid fasting. It delivers the greatest level of therapeutic benefit physically and in a short period of time, as detox occurs more quickly. But a water fast can be more difficult to commit to for the beginner. Only water is consumed during this fast. No other liquids or solid foods.

DRY FASTING

Also known as Absolute Fast, Black Fast, and Hebrew Fast. The most extreme of the types of fasting, dry fasting has spiritual roots, and consists of foregoing food and water for short periods. Not recommended for beginners or necessarily recommended in general to the average person based upon a variety of factors such as activities of daily living, space for extensive rest, and adequate resources to have in place in preparation for recovery.

CHAPTER 4

Preparing To Fast

When preparing to fast, there are many things that will race through your mind such as, the type of fast you want to do, if you have everything prepared to help you recover from your fast, possible events or activities you have coming up, should you tell anyone you're fasting, ways you can manage stress, and if your energy will be decreased during the day, among other concerns. All these concerns are important, otherwise, they would not cross your mind. However, how you prepare for your fast will help deter and alleviate many of these concerns. It is crucial to first begin to practice fasting/abstaining from certain harmful items. This will help reduce cravings and temptations towards many items while also helping to build up the tolerance your body will need (physically and mentally) while fasting. Below you will find some helpful tips on ways to prepare for your fast so that you will effectively work through a fast and be able to experience the many benefits that fasting has to offer.

1). Have a plan for how you will recover and transition out of your fast. Your plan should involve one transition day for every three days that you have fasted for ("3:1 Ratio"; we'll go more in detail about the 3:1 Ratio later on), a list of certain foods you will consume as you build back up to more solid foods and meals, and a plan to stick to consuming healthier foods after your fast so you can continue on with your journey of living a healthier lifestyle. Creating a list of fruits, vegetables, herbs, and grains will help map out what you will want to consume and also determine how much you may need upon completing your fast or items you'll need during your fast. Please reference the Dr. Sebi Nutritional Guide for a list of natural foods that help provide the most nourishment for our bodies with the least amount of items containing materials detrimental to our health.

2). Drastically lighten up your toxic load and accumulation. Alcohol, liquor, coffee, cigarettes, refined sugars, fast foods, saturated fats, dairy products, meat, poultry, seafood, wheat, etc. All of these items represent additional obstacles in the healing process. It is best to eliminate these from your diet altogether, but particularly when preparing for a fast. Loading up on toxins while preparing for a process such as fasting (which works to remove toxins and waste materials) is counterproductive. While we should not consume the items listed, it is of most importance to do so when preparing for a fast so that your fasting process can be effective. If you have difficulty removing any of these items when preparing to fast, you will only experience more difficulty restraining from these same foods during your fast and it would be in your best interest to shift your focus on consuming more healthy foods at this time and plan to fast at a later date.

After attempting to digest and absorb the necessary minerals that it needs, the body will often store away anything that it does not recognize which turns into fat. The body is attempting to process all the material that is consumed and while making sure to dissect and hold onto what it needs; this can be at its' own detriment. The body will store away harmful substances trying to break them down in order to be expelled from the body, but consistent accumulation of toxins creates an overloaded system in which these substances will turn into fat, spill over into the bloodstream, get into the bones, and pretty much find a hiding space to get into for the moment while trying to recruit more substances to feed on for its' survival, which most commonly comes in the form of food cravings.

3). Another obstacle or hindrance to work on removing when preparing for fasting is STRESS. Just seeing the word stress in all capitals may have triggered some emotions within yourself. Stress triggers your body to release stress-hormones into your system. While these hormones can provide a type of adrenaline rush to win a race or meet a deadline on a project, when released in large amounts repeatedly, they create toxins within the body and slow down detoxification enzymes in the liver and kidneys. The liver is the primary detoxifying organ in the body, along with the kidneys, lungs, and the skin. Causing backup for the detoxifying organs will prevent the body from removing toxins you wish to get rid of while preparing for and upon completing a fast.

Another reason to work on reducing your stress prior to and during your fast is because the body creates salt when it is under constant or unprovoked stress. Salt (sodium-chloride) dehydrates the body. Sodium-chloride is present in most processed foods which typically leads to one feeling thirsty afterwards, headaches, feelings of fatigue, or bruising easily, because the body is becoming dehydrated. Imagine fasting, eating relatively well, and drinking water but still feeling dehydrated and experiencing these symptoms. This will not make for a pleasant fasting experience or keep you motivated to eat well afterwards.

The body needs to REMAIN hydrated; not just to get hydrated regularly. Getting our hydration comes from the water we drink, but also from the fresh fruits and vegetables that we eat. Water is made of H2O which involves two Hydrogen atoms and one Oxygen atom. Hydrogen-rich foods and Oxygen-rich foods are crucial to our health and survival.

Hydrogen and Oxygen are two of the most crucial elements we need to survive. The body also must stay hydrated to properly absorb all the many benefits that it consumes. When a single cell is deprived of oxygen up to 30% of its' capacity, this promotes cell erosion, in addition to cells duplicating abnormally as their requirements (minerals) are left unfulfilled. This abnormal fashion in which those cells replicate is referred to as, "Abnormal Cell Growth", or more commonly known as the condition we know as "Cancer".

A nucleus of an atom can only hold two electrons (electrons are electrical charges for the cells) in the 1st valance and eight in the remainder valances (outer shells of an electron). When dealing with stress, we most often get upset or frustrated. When we get upset or frustrated (heat rises in the body) this causes the Sodium in the body (Na) molecule to throw an electron off of its structure in an attempt to function by removing any "baggage" or hindrances. This makes it unstable and causes it to create a bond with whatever is compatible with it in its current state (this is called "Covalent Bonding"). In this case, the Sodium molecule is now compatible with the element Chlorine (Cl) because Chlorine produces "free" electrons to the body. Chlorine gives off free electrons to other elements in the body in case they need any as we use our energy in different ways throughout our daily lives.

Now you have Na + Cl which is "NaCl" which creates Sodium Chloride aka "Salt".

We can eat right but if we are around people who get us upset or situations that make us upset and frustrated, we will continue to accumulate salt within the body. These people and situations will create the same thing we are looking to escape from.

Fasting and preparing for fasting under these conditions will become detrimental to your health. While not eating or consuming much, the last thing our bodies need is to become dehydrated. This would not create an enjoyable experience and will not adequately address the primary needs a person hopes to address by fasting.

Use these steps while preparing to fast as these same steps will be necessary for a healthy lifestyle outside of fasting. As you will see, Fasting is not only about physically removing toxins from the body, but about emotionally and spiritually cleaning the body, the mind, and the soul together as one.

CHAPTER 5

How Long To Fast

Give careful consideration when deciding how long to fast. If you have never fasted before, a commitment of a day or less is easier to accomplish and will familiarize you with the process. Use this first experience to learn what your body's particular reactions are. Every body is unique. You need to learn about yours. Length of time for a fast should always be the length that is right for you at the time. Remain flexible. Of course, you will have a goal in mind when you begin, but don't be too inflexible to end the fast should your body signal signs of difficulty.

Be careful not to fast too frequently. Allow your body sufficient time to rebuild its nutritional reserves. Recommended fasting times for regular, occasional maintenance and rebalancing are one day per week and/or 3 days per month and/or around 36-52 days yearly. As you can see, this is close to 1-2 months of fasting for the year! Now, this fasting recommendation is just prolonged fasting from what you are typically use to. However, you can always push through with a full day (24 hour) fast a few times per month throughout the year and those days do add up. You may also choose to do an Intermittent Fasting method year-round and change the time gap in which you consume solid foods based on your personal schedule.

Whichever you choose to do, making fasting a part of your regular lifestyle, shifts how you view your relationship with what you consume. You will no longer eat "just because". What you eat and when you eat will come with intention. This will not only make it simpler to eat while going forward, but extend the quantity and quality of your life by needing less maintenance throughout your lifespan. Gradual and scheduled maintenance beats damage control any day.

For those who wish to do an extended fast, keep in mind that you cannot fast for 5 or 10 days if you do not first begin fasting for 1 day. Take it one day at a time regardless of your goal and maintain an accurate assessment of how you are doing, particularly keeping in the mind the type of fast you are doing. The most important thing is to get started.

If you are doing a liquid fast and feel fatigued or have a headache, this may be a signal to drink some more liquids. However, if you are doing a dry fast and begin to feel fatigued or have a headache, you should use this as an opportunity to break this particular fast and begin to consume some liquids to avoid any complications or potentially harmful effects that you can experience. In this scenario, you may transition from a dry fast to a liquid fast, and eventually work your way up towards partial or intermittent fasting at this time.

You may do this at any point and over time, with experience, you will further understand your body and your personal tolerance to fasting and slowly build up your tolerance for the future.

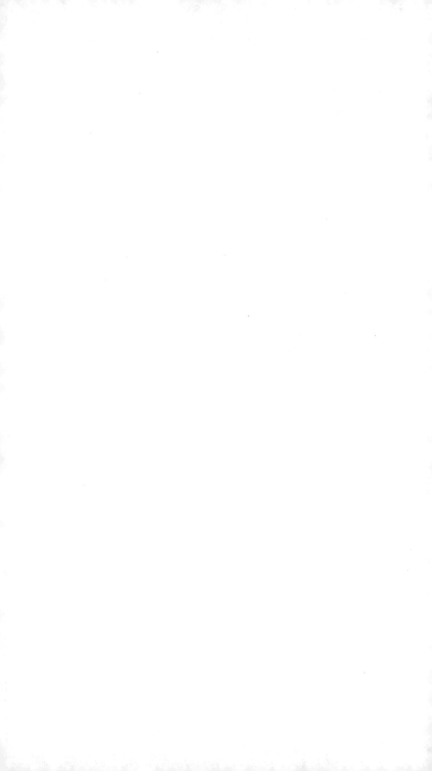

CHAPTER 6

Using Sleep To Your Advantage

The average person typically will start their clock upon awakening and fit everything in by the time they go back to sleep. However, our bodies remain awake and alert if we are alive and breathing. There is still work to do while one is asleep. When we go to sleep our bodies are naturally in a fasting state because we are abstaining ourselves from eating. This is the time when our bodies are healing and rebuilding.

Society has taught us to wake up and eat before our bodies are fully awake and alert enough to absorb anything. The Standard American Diet (SAD) which has become a more standard global diet, promotes a breakfast to consist of flesh, starch, mucus, and acid (potatoes, bacon, eggs, pancakes, and flavored chemical juices). These foods clog the arteries and intestines as well as promote mucus proliferation and cellular erosion. This way of eating is not helping us but only pushing us closer to disease and illness. Even delaying your consumption of these items through fasting will make a world of difference; literally. A Standard American Diet will only promote standard American diseases and conditions (diabetes, cancer, high blood pressure, dementia, asthma).

First and foremost, you must work to not hinder your sleep by consuming things difficult to digest such as the foods listed above, eating late at night, or even not allowing yourself to power down as you approach a time you wish to sleep. Eating later at night or shortly prior to sleeping, your internal organs will be processing and digesting everything still while you are trying to rest. This process will either wake you up several times throughout the time you are asleep, create discomfort, or leave you feeling fatigued and tired upon awakening since your body will still be working full-time while attempting to rest, repair, and recover.

We have constructed our time to start and end each day within a certain time range. We must expand how we view our time and how it is constructed within our daily lives. This is where fasting can help you make positive use of the time you are not capturing. When you make intentional use of your time you feel more fulfilled. Feelings such worry, fear, and anger begin to diminish, you become more relaxed and can conserve the energy that you created which is building inside of you.

Sleep is about fasting. Every time we go to sleep and shut the digestive system down the body automatically goes into repair. The more waste and toxins to process in the body, the more sleep is required. The less waste and toxins needed to process in the body, the less sleep is needed. Sleep is the reparation period where the body breaks down the cells it does not need and works to rebuild new cells. If you are not able to get adequate rest due to your daily schedule (having children to care for, waking up early for work, working long hours), you will experience symptoms such as fatigue, headaches, body pains, memory impairment, as well as trigger many mental health conditions. This is where fasting helps to provide relief as you work towards a healthier lifestyle.

Just because we use the bathroom and eliminate waste somewhat regularly does not mean we do not have any mucus stuck in our organs and the buildup of toxins from all the years of eating junk. This buildup of waste creates a toxic environment which leads to illness. While sleeping, our bodies begin the restoration process but far too often do not get enough time to commit to any lasting or noticeable effects due to regular consumption of foods (especially harmful ones). Imagine cooking your favorite meal and leaving it uncovered on the stove for a few days or just overnight. It is going to begin to rot and not be something you would want to consume because it is beginning to spoil and become fermented. Now imagine this process happening in your precious body for several years with no cleaning. We clean our houses, we clean our cars, we clean our jewelry, but very few realize the importance of cleaning the body. Cleansing and repairing the body is the physical manifestation that fasting represents. We can create this experience whenever we are sleeping and getting quality rest.

Being mindful of the hours we are asleep as being a part of our fasting schedule, getting quality sleep becomes a priority. Quality sleep not only helps you wake up feeling rested, but can increase cognitive abilities, help you feel more energized, and increase your motivation to work towards your goals, thus, adding to the overall quality of your life.

Melatonin is often referred to as the natural "sleep chemical" within the body. Not to be confused with "Serotonin", which is one of the, many the "happy chemicals" within the body, Melatonin is actually a hormone that is released naturally within the body on a daily schedule to help promote sleep. When this hormone is released, you may feel drowsy, begin yawning, and feel sleepy.

There are many foods which contain Melatonin and/ or promote a release of Melatonin in our bodies that we can consume to promote this experience. For example, many fruits such as bananas and cherries, leafy green vegetables, and many grains and nuts contain Melatonin and/or promote our body's ability to produce and hold onto Melatonin. Consuming these foods are often recommended to help those who have difficulty getting quality sleep. These foods will not necessarily cause you to feel tired or go to sleep if you eat them during the day. The body simply stores away the Melatonin until the body is triggered to get some rest, and this chemical is now released to help support getting quality rest. This is the importance of consuming these items regularly so that you have an adequate amount stored away in your body's reserves, particularly when fasting or preparing for a fast.

While fasting, the body can produce Melatonin more regularly in accordance with our Circadian Rhythm. A "Circadian Rhythm" is a natural, internal process that regulates the sleep-wake cycle. This also includes our body's ability to regulate temperature, blood temperature, and alertness. When fasting, we can regulate our body's working conditions and functions, which in turn, promotes Melatonin production as needed.

Being able to rely on regular quality sleep, fasting becomes easier and helps directly contribute to overall lifestyle changes we wish to work towards. As we feel more rested, we can make more positive choices regarding our health and continue to take larger steps towards improving our health and wellness.

As you adjust to regularly fasting, you will notice that six to eight hours of quality sleep may feel much better than eight or more hours of interrupted sleep. Gaining more quality sleep by having a regular fasting regimen can very well be the missing link you need to achieve many of your personal health and lifestyle goals.

CHAPTER 7

Should I Exercise While Fasting?

Resting is particularly important during the fasting stage. Many will want to work out and exercise during this time, but when fasting you have to allow the body to rest in order for it to do what it's intended to do, which is heal itself. Doing a regular fasting routine or method such as Intermittent Fasting will be fine but anything more than that, or on days you may plan for a full twenty-four hour fast, you will want to avoid physical exercise.

Most of us live hectic lives, so you may not be able to go on vacation somewhere to just relax while fasting. Understanding and analyzing your situation will be vital in your approach to healing. Whatever you must do for your livelihood will be fine, but other than that, rest and taking it easy every chance you get is crucial. At most, the average person should do some brisk walking, stretching, maybe a Yoga class or some other structured class that involves light to moderate physical activity.

Working out regularly while fasting puts a hindrance on your healing process. Instead of the focus being on cleansing or detoxing, now the body must take that energy to account for the additional workload that you are creating during your workout. Also, this depletes a lot of the nutrition you are taking in daily, leaving you to feel exhausted and wondering how much longer you can sustain your fast. Exercising and burning calories can lead to many food cravings and push you more towards breaking your fast than working to prolong your fast.

If you are doing something such as a 24hr fast or doing Intermittent Fasting regularly, it is not necessary to stop or delay your typical training regimen. However, if you are planning to do a longer than normal fast for your body, consider decreasing the intensity of your workout and/or the number of sets you do to allow your body to adjust. If you exercise regularly, you will typically be aware of your limitations and ways to push yourself. You want to remain proactive with how you approach your exercise regime while fasting so that you do not have to take additional time to recover.

Many people do "fasted cardio" where they will do some light to moderate cardio prior to their first meal to help burn excess fat and/or cardio. Anyone who goes running or jogging first thing in the morning is essentially doing fasted cardio however, not everyone is following a fasting regimen. Those who have a fasting schedule, their cardio will have a specific schedule as well.

So, while fasting, yes you can exercise; it would just be more beneficial if you chose not to or done very minimally. You do want to be mindful of your tolerance and experience with exercise. Pushing yourself more than your body may be prepared for while fasting can cause you to break your fast which you do not want to be forced into doing.

Your best bet would be to engage in low to moderate training of any kind while also exploring other forms of training. You could join in on a Yoga class, a Boxing and/or Kickboxing class, try out some form of Martial Art or self-defense. Any structured class involving exercise, instructors and participants are generally disciplined and can become a support network for you while you are fasting.

You can get some experience while pursuing a new interest while also learning more about other ways of training. Calisthenics (body weight) exercises are also a great form of exercise that will prevent you from overexerting yourself during a workout because you are using your own body weight for movement when training certain muscle groups.

As you gain more experience with fasting, you will grasp a better understanding of your body and its current limitations. You may get to a point where you can do any fasting method while pushing yourself physically while exercising. You just should not experiment with this as you get use to fasting. Like anything else, it takes regular practice and you will want to be able to increase your tolerance over time so your body can properly adjust.

CHAPTER 8

Sample Fasting Routines vs Cleansing and Detoxing

Fasting as you can already tell, is simple. But just because it is simple, does not mean that it is easy. You want to organize routines for what you can do to make this process much easier. There are, however, distinct differences between Fasting, Cleansing, and Detoxing, which are terms often used interchangeably.

When doing a Cleanse, you are focused mostly on your gut health and helping the digestive system work without additional hindrances. The "Gut" is a large piece of the immune system connecting to the colon. You are essentially cleansing toxins that negatively impact your body's response systems that clean out waste materials. Occasionally you may lose some weight, but more often than not, it is what comes after a cleanse (diet/lifestyle) that create any weight loss if that is your goal. When most people do a Cleanse, all they are doing is consuming foods (mostly in liquid form) that are easy to digest at once so the body can become nourished from those foods and by default, not seek out other foods to consume. This frees up the digestive tract of additional work to do and allows it to regain its energy and work towards functioning more properly. Cleansing is supported by also removing or refraining from eating foods difficult to digest such as eggs, meat, dairy, gluten, soy, refined sugars, processed foods, and/or alcohol. A person becomes accustomed to not consuming these foods for nourishment, and can then work in healthier alternatives than they are used to consuming.

Detoxing, on the other hand, has to do with addressing any difficulty the detoxifying organs (liver, kidneys, lungs, and skin) are having with removing waste from the body. Nothing else takes place during a Detox. Anyone who tries to sell or promote a Detox for the other internal organs, or promotes a Detox that does not focus primarily on the liver and/or kidneys, are just trying to take your money. Or they could be just using the wrong word since "Detox" and "Cleanse" are words often used interchangeably. The liver and kidneys work with other organs to keep the rest of your body detoxified, but sometimes they need a little boost. You can however, provide a cleanse targeting the Colon as well as removing parasites from the body as these two will allow the kidneys and liver to detox excess waste more efficiently which helps to also clean this section of the body. Cleaning the Colon and/or doing a Detox focused on removing parasites from the body should only be done sparingly.

As with cleansing, when you Detox, you want to cut out certain foods like refined sugars, alcohol, and other processed foods. After you have eliminated these items, it is best to incorporate foods that help strengthen the liver and kidneys during this time so they can work more effectively going forward.

Fasting, is different than a Cleanse and a Detox because it is only about giving your internal organs (particularly your digestive system) a much-needed break, which promotes the self-healing processes our bodies were born with.

To provide a better picture of the differences between a Cleanse, a Detox, and Fasting, think about cleaning your home. A Cleanse would be dusting off your furniture, and wiping down tables. A Detox would involve a need for a home inspection while inviting specific tradesmen to come and address specific needs you may have (plumbing issue, fixing some electrical work, etc). While Fasting, would be the equivalent of rearranging furniture along with some deep cleaning, while imagining updates you can plan for in the future.

Most Common Fasting Routines

Fasting For Health Chart	
Dry Fast	Can be completed a few times a year. Helps reset metabolism by improving detoxification process.
3-5 Day Water Fast	Best used for preventative measures.
36-48 Hour Water Fast	Helps the body reach in for its reserves for nourishment and work to repair the body.
Autophagy	Minimum of 5 days out of each month, autophagy is necessary to help maintain homeostasis as the body work on repairing the body.
24-Hour, OMAD *OMAD = "One Meal A Day"	Minimum 3-4 days each month helps to promote natural Ketosis and losing weight while processing toxins for their removal.
Intermittent Fasting	Daily 13-16hr fast between meals. Baseline for general health, weight loss, mental clarity, and energy.

As you can see from the chart, Intermittent Fasting is something you can do daily if you choose. The other fasting methods in this chart are to be done somewhat sparingly. As you get use to fasting, doing a full day (24hr) fast becomes more manageable. Moving on from this, doing several days on just liquids becomes a way to test your tolerance until you eventually can set a goal for a dry fast or water fast a few times a year. As stated earlier, the days you fast will add up over time.

Intermittent Fasting

6 Types of Intermittent Fasting	
16/8	16-hour fast each day with an 8-hour time period to consume solid foods. Water is accepted outside of the 16-hour fasting period. This is the most popular method of Intermittent Fasting.
5/2	Fast for 2 full days each week. This may include the 16:8 method at first but is to be used as a tool to help prepare the body and mind for prolonged fasting.
Eat-Stop-Eat	Fast for 24-hours once or twice per week.
Alternate Day Fasting	Fast every other day.
Warrior Diet	Fast during the day followed by one larger meal for dinner.
Spontaneous Meal Skipping	Skip meals when convenient (either breakfast or dinner) that coincides with your sleep schedule to make your fasting period easier to accomplish.

Intermittent Fasting is by far the most common fasting method as you can structure it into you day in a variety of ways. The word "intermittent" refers to occurring at irregular intervals as this fasting method will appear irregular to your current standard of consuming items during the day.

When Intermittent Fasting, 16:8 is the goal, but if you choose Alternate Day Fasting or the 5:2 schedule, you will want to generally keep your calories low on days that you fast. Counting calories is not always an enjoyable way towards living a healthier lifestyle, but by eating foods low in calories (mostly fruits, certain vegetables, and herbal teas) on days that you choose to fast, this will in turn, keep your calorie count low and help you stay around the recommended calories often needed while fasting.

The main thing is to give your body much time to rest. Calories are units of energy. When we eat, we use these calories to provide us with energy. When we are fasting, we do not want to remain regularly active, which is why the calories should also be low to not promote or encourage us to become very active during this time period of healing; although you will notice an increase in energy and alertness from removing fatigue, headaches, and other hindrances you may experience in your daily life.

Intermittent Fasting can be done regularly, but you do want to remain mindful of how your body responds to any or all the following methods, and slowly incorporate a fasting routine for yourself based on your current needs.

The 16/8 Method							
	Day 1	Day 2	Day 3	Day 4	Day 5	Day 6	Day 7
Midnight	Fast	Fast	Fast	Fast	Fast	Fast	Fast
4am	Fast	Fast	Fast	Fast	Fast	Fast	Fast
8am	Fast	Fast	Fast	Fast	Fast	Fast	Fast
12pm	First Meal	First Meal	First Meal	First Meal	First Meal	First Meal	First Meal
4pm	Last Meal By 8pm	Last Meal By 8pm	Last Meal By 8pm	Last Meal By 8pm	Last Meal By 8pm	Last Meal By 8pm	Last Meal By 8pm
8pm	Fast	Fast	Fast	Fast	Fast	Fast	Fast
Midnight	Fast	Fast	Fast	Fast	Fast	Fast	Fast

Here is the typical standard for Intermittent Fasting.

Many will have to work their way up to this mode, while others can jump right into it. You will want to practice doing one day or so out of the week to get a feel for this method at first. You want to see how this routine settles into your lifestyle and adequately planning out items you will eat as you break your fast.

Not everyone's schedule will be as clear as the image above, but the time periods should remain the same. People work various jobs and different shifts, but if you can structure your fasting schedule in accordance with your sleep schedule and keep the general 16:8 schedule, then you are Intermittent Fasting!

The 5:2 Diet						
Day 1	Day 2	Day 3	Day 4	Day 5	Day 6	Day 7
Eats Normally	Women: 600 Calories Men: 500 Calories	Eats Normally	Eats Normally	Women: 600 Calories Men: 500 Calories	Eats Normally	Eats Normally

The 5:2 Diet is also a form of Intermittent Fasting as you are just not fasting continuously each day. This method is great for beginners who can choose a day of the week that they are the least active and choose to fast. This method fits in well for those who often overindulge and want to train themselves into limiting

how much they intake a few days a week. This method can be used as a checkpoint while working towards a 16:8 schedule.

Eat-Stop-Eat						
Day 1	Day 2	Day 3	Day 4	Day 5	Day 6	Day 7
Eats Normally	24-Hour Fast	Eats Normally	Eats Normally	24-Hour Fast	Eats Normally	Eats Normally

Eat-Stop-Eat involves a full 24-hour fast once or twice a week. You will want to eat relatively normally during this time period but also making some room for dietary and lifestyle adjustments. The most common way this fast is completed is by starting your fast after eating dinner and carrying this out until you have dinner the following day. You can drink liquids during each 24-hour fast, but no solid foods are permitted. You also want to plan for a day to fast after every 2-3 days to help your body build up its reserves that it will rely on while fasting using this method.

Alternate Day Fasting						
Day 1	Day 2	Day 3	Day 4	Day 5	Day 6	Day 7
Eats Normally	24-Hour Fast Or Eat only a few hundred calories	Eats Normally	24-Hour Fast Or Eat only a few hundred calories	Eats Normally	24-Hour Fast Or Eat only a few hundred calories	Eats Normally

The next step from the 5:2 method and Eat-Stop-Eat method is Alternate Day Fasting. This method you simply add a third day of fasting that involves low calories or choose to fast completely for an entire 24-hour time period. A large part of the 24-hour time period is covered while sleeping. It is important that your diet consists of foods that provide adequate nutrition on your non-fasting days because if you are fasting for an extended period of time several days per week, you want to make sure that the rest of your week you are being properly nourished to limit difficulties while fasting.

If you feel you are starving or depriving yourself on your fasting days, then you are not properly nourishing your body on your non-fasting days. You may want to work in a green smoothie or juice in the mornings on your normal eating days to provide additional nourishment to your body as you adjust to fasting.

Spontaneous Meal Skipping						
Day 1	Day 2	Day 3	Day 4	Day 5	Day 6	Day 7
Breakfast	*Skipped Meal*	Breakfast	Breakfast	Breakfast	Breakfast	Breakfast
Lunch	Lunch	Lunch	Lunch	Lunch	Lunch	Lunch
Dinner	Dinner	Dinner	Dinner	*Skipped Meal*	Dinner	Dinner

Spontaneous Meal Skipping is often what we all do at some point. We often skip lunch if we are busy at work, go to bed early and skip dinner, or just are not hungry during a certain time of day and do not eat. The method, however, calls for planning out skipping a meal prior to, or after sleeping so that you have (at least) two days where you scheduled in a fast. This method is a beginner method to introduce yourself to fasting while helping to feel the positive benefits that fasting can provide for your health.

You will want to get your body accustomed to not consuming several meals a day out of habit. Planning out a meal you will skip will give you time to prepare for fasting mentally and physically until this becomes more of a regular habit. You will want to skip either breakfast or dinner, so it connects to your sleeping schedule.

When Spontaneous Meal Skipping, you want to be cautious to avoid overindulging on days you are not fasting, although this may happen at first. You simply want to plan when you will fast so that you can introduce healthier foods into your lifestyle as they will promote recovery and nourishment. This includes but is not limited to fruit smoothies and juices, herbal teas, soups, and plant-based meals.

	Day 1	Day 2	Day 3	Day 4	Day 5	Day 6	Day 7
				The Warrior Diet			
Midnight	Fast	Fast	Fast	Fast	Fast	Fast	Fast
4am	Fast	Fast	Fast	Fast	Fast	Fast	Fast
8am	Eat small amount of fruits and vegetables	Eat small amount of fruits and vegetables	Eat small amount of fruits and vegetables	Eat small amount of fruits and vegetables	Eat small amount of fruits and vegetables	Eat small amount of fruits and vegetables	Eat small amount of fruits and vegetables
12pm	Eat small amount of fruits and vegetables	Eat small amount of fruits and vegetables	Eat small amount of fruits and vegetables	Eat small amount of fruits and vegetables	Eat small amount of fruits and vegetables	Eat small amount of fruits and vegetables	Eat small amount of fruits and vegetables
4pm	Eat Large Meal	Eat Large Meal	Eat Large Meal	Eat Large Meal	Eat Large Meal	Eat Large Meal	Eat Large Meal
8pm	Fast	Fast	Fast	Fast	Fast	Fast	Fast
Midnight	Fast	Fast	Fast	Fast	Fast	Fast	Fast

The Warrior diet is for those who have built up a tolerance for fasting. This fasting method also serves well for those looking to lose weight. We have all had days where we have snacked on various foods during the day and planned for a larger meal at night. What makes the Warrior Diet different, is the intention that is set while following this schedule daily.

More fresh fruits and vegetables are to be introduced

(or re-introduced) to the body during this method. The exact hours may be different for you than they are in the image above, but the concept is the same: snacking on foods during the day while preparing for a larger meal in the evening.

As with any plan, you want to incorporate as many foods that are healthier than your typical lifestyle consists of. Planning only one meal a day takes an incredible amount of pressure off of your plate (literally) with the time you save to prepare and cook multiple meals even if for a short period of time when fasting. Some may choose to make this method a more consistent lifestyle change and follow this method for an extended period of time.

Many often stick to this particular fasting method prior to adjusting to a liquid, water, or dry fast. The Warrior Diet helps to set the intention of consuming foods that are beneficial to your health and create a stronger relationship with the foods you consume as you more directly experience their benefits as you work towards an overall healthier lifestyle.

Liquid and Water Fasting

Liquid Fasting consists of Water, Juices, Smoothies, Herbal Teas, and even some Soups. During a Liquid Fast, you are simply replacing your solid foods with liquids. Liquid fasting is great way to pack in many of the essential minerals that we need for our survival. You can combine a wide variety of fruits and vegetables that you ordinarily would not put together to eat, but receive the many benefits that these items contain. If you are already use to eating fruits and vegetables, this will put you at an advantage as you'll have a better grasp of what foods to combine, how certain items taste together, and will understand others things such as texture, how much juice you may get out of some foods, and the primary and secondary benefits many fruits and vegetables have to offer. A major benefit of doing a Liquid Fast or Water Fast, is that you can consume these substances all day starting and ending at any time. This helps to avoid feeling deprived of anything or must mentally and physically work through any wait periods during the day.

You will want to already become use to making juices and smoothies prior to beginning a liquid fast as you will want to have experience mixing certain fruits and vegetables, while also understanding how much liquid you will be able to get from particular fruits and vegetables. This is important because you want to have an adequate amount of liquids available at your disposal without feeling as if your underachieving or not consuming enough during your liquid fast.

You may end up getting more nourishment from liquid fasting than with your typical diet at times. This is due to the increased amount of fresh fruits and vegetables you use to make your smoothies and juices. It takes an adequate amount of fruits and vegetables to make several full servings to drink throughout the day in addition to water. With the added nourishment, you may also find it easier to recover from a liquid fast without overindulging once you have completed your fast.

Many herbs also contain more minerals and nutrients than some whole foods do. Drinking herbal teas daily will help to further enhance the healing properties of fasting. Herbs are naturally healing as they contain many natural chemicals that help to prevent inflammation and illness or disease. Other herbs work specifically to address the primary symptoms of many diseases and help the body absorb the necessary minerals and nutrients it consumes. Including herbal teas into your liquid fast will allow your body to make up for any minerals it may be deficient in, while also providing your body with more healing properties to help repair and revitalize any areas in need within your body. This will directly help to improve the digestive tract, boost your immune system, and clean out much of the waste that may remain in your body.

You may experience short term weight loss during a liquid fast, but often, it is due to the body getting rid of what it does not need. As you consume more liquids, the detoxifying organs (liver, kidneys, lungs, and skin) can spend more time breaking down any accumulation of toxins and materials that you may have in your body, as it does not have to break down any solids. The liquids you will be consuming, allows the body to filter out things more regularly and work more on absorbing the many benefits that juices, smoothies, teas, and soups have to offer. Liquid Fasting is typically only a few days on average but can be extended for a full week, or longer.

Here are some examples of a 3-Day, 4-day, and 5-Day Liquid Fast. It should be noted with precaution that, anything close to one full week (7 days) on a liquid fast, you will want to be able to do at least a 4-5 day liquid fast with minimal discomfort before attempting a 7 day or longer liquid fast.

3 Day Liquid Fast

Morning:

2 teaspoons of Key Lime Juice
1 tablespoon of Tahini Butter
1 Banana
1 Cup of Raspberries
¼ Cup of Kale
1 Tablespoon of Hemp seeds
1 Cup of Spring Water

Lunch:

1 Cucumber
1 Cup of Kale Leaves
1 Key Lime (peeled)
½ Green Apple
1.5 Cups of Walnut Milk
1 Cup of Watermelon

Dinner:

1 Cup of Blueberries
½ Cup of Mango
1 Cup of Kale
¼ Avocado
1 teaspoon of Key Lime Juice
¼ teaspoon of Cayenne Pepper
1.5 Cups of Coconut Water

You can drink water throughout the day as well to remain hydrated. You can also make larger servings as well, if everything is in proportion to the recipe listed.

4-Day Liquid Fast

	Breakfast	Lunch	Dinner
Day 1	2 Apples 1 Cucumber 1 Cup of Blueberries 2 Cups of Grapes 2 Kale Leaves 1 teaspoon of Ginger	2 Apples 1 Orange 1 Handful of Dandelion Greens 1 Cup of Mango 4 Kale Leaves Small pinch of Mint	2 Kale Leaves 1 Handful of Amaranth Greens 2 Peeled Key Limes 1 teaspoon of Ginger Half Handful of Basil
Day 2	2 Apples 1 Cup of Blueberries 2 Kale Leaves 1 Cup of Blackberries 1 Peeled Key Lime 1 Cup of Fresh Orange Juice	2 Apples 1 Cucumber 1 Handful of Turnip Greens 1 Pear 1 Cup of Mixed Berries	2 Cucumbers 2 Kale Leaves 3 Pears 2 Peeled Key Limes
Day 3	2 Apples 2 Oranges 1 Cup of Blackberries 1 Cup of Coconut Water Half Handful of Cilantro	2 Apples 1 Red Pepper (Chopped) 2 Tomatoes (remove seeds) ½ Jalapeno Pepper Small Handful of Cilantro	3 Cucumbers 2 Kale Leaves 3 Pears 2 Peels Key Limes

Day 4	2 Oranges 1 Cup of Mango 2 Bananas 1 Peeled Key Lime Small amount of Fresh Mint	1 Apple 1 Cucumber 1 Small Handful of Basil 1 Pear 2 teaspoons of Ginger	1 Apple 2 Cups of Mango 3 Pears 1 tablespoon of Ginger

All of the items listed for each "meal" are to be juiced or blended together to create a smoothie.

5-Day Liquid Fast

Day 1	Day 2	Day 3	Day 4	Day 5
(8am) 28oz of Warm Water w. Key Limes	(8am) 28oz Warm Water w/ Key Limes	(8am) 28oz Water w/Key Limes	(8am) 28oz Water w/Key Limes	(8am) 32oz Water w/Key Limes
(9am) 20 oz Green Drink	(9am) 12oz of Orange Drink	(9am) 20oz Green Drink	(9am) 20oz Green Drink	(9am) 20oz Green Drink
(10am) 16oz Water	(10am) 16oz Water	(10am) 16oz Water)	(10am) 32oz Water)	(12pm) 16oz Water
(12pm) 16 oz Red Drink	(11am) 22oz of Green Drink	(11am) 16oz Green Drink	(12pm) 16oz Green Drink	(1pm) 16oz Green Drink
(1pm) 12oz Coconut Water	(12pm) 16oz Water	(12pm) 16oz Water	(3pm) 16oz Blood Cleanser Tea	(3pm) Lung Support Tea
(3pm) 8oz Red Drink	(2pm)16oz Water	(1pm) 16oz Green Drink	(4pm) 16oz Green Drink	(4pm) 16oz Water
(4pm) 16oz Water	(4pm) 20oz Green Drink	(3pm) 32oz Peppermint Tea)	(6pm) 16oz water	(6pm) 16oz Green Drink
(6pm) 16oz Green Drink	(5pm) 16oz Water	(5pm) 16oz Water	(7pm) 32oz Ginger Tea	(8pm) 32oz Ginger Tea
(730pm) 28oz Ginger Tea	(6pm) 16oz Water	(6pm) 16oz Green Drink		
	(7pm) 16oz Green Drink (730pm)	(7pm) 16oz Water	*Blood Cleanser Tea Consists of: Sarsaparilla, Burdock, and Guaco.	*Lung Support Tea Consists of: Elderberry, Mullein, Dandelion Root, Palo Guaco, and Wild Cherry Bark.
*Green Drink Consists of: Kale, Cucumber, Green Apples, and Ginger Root.	8oz Colon Cleanse Tea	(8pm) 32oz Ginger Tea		
**Make enough for Day 1 and 2 (36oz total)	(8pm) 16oz Water			
*Red Drink Consists of: Apples, Raspberries, Cherries, Pears, Dandelion Greens, and Cucumber.	*Orange Drink Consists of: Oranges, Mango, Burro Banana, and Ginger Root.			
	*Colon Cleanse Tea Consists of: Cascara Sagrada, Black Walnut, and Rhubarb Root.			

Green Drink: 2 Green Apples, 1 Cucumber, Large Handful of Kale, and 1 inch of Ginger Root.

Red Drink: 2 Apples, 2 Cups of Raspberries, ¾ Cup of Cherries (seeded, remove seeds), 2 Pears, 1 Small handful of Dandelion Greens, and 2.5 Cups of Watermelon

Orange Drink: 3 Oranges, 2 Mangoes, 2 Burro Bananas, and 1 inch of Ginger Root.

With any of these drinks, you are free to use other ingredients as well. These are just to start you off with basic drinks that will meet the recommended ounces for each drink on a daily basis. You do not want to shortchange yourself or not have an adequate amount to drink while on a liquid fast. It will also be best to have more available than what your need. You can mix up the drinks for each day as well based upon what items you have at your disposal. The colors of each drink (Green, Red, and Orange) are not chosen to just mix up the variety of foods, they are chosen due to certain colors of natural foods provide particular benefits to the body which are of most importance while fasting.

The Green drink contains Chlorophyll and Folate which help to build healthy cells and remove carcinogens. The primary goal for optimum health and longevity is to feed your cells while removing carcinogens (cancer-causing items). Green drinks are very popular for these two reasons and are the result of leafy green vegetables that remain a staple in any healthy lifestyle.

The Orange drink contains Beta-Carotene which work to boost the immune system. As your body processes items it is working to remove and other items to absorb, the last thing you want is your immune system to be unprepared and respond rapidly, leading to you developing a sickness or fever, or end up experiencing headaches and fatigue.

The Red drink contains antioxidants that you want in your system to help kill and bacteria and protect your cells during this time.

Other Items Listed In This 5-Day Liquid Fast:

Colon Cleanse Tea: 1 teaspoon of Cascara Sagrada, ½ teaspoon of Black Walnut, and 1 teaspoon of Rhubarb Root for about 10-12oz of tea. This tea is very bitter. But you want this tea to be bitter so that it can break down what is not needed in the body. If this tea is too difficult for you to adjust to, you can always search for these herbs or colon cleanses available in capsule form. You will want to try this tea prior to fasting to identify which option will be best for you during your liquid fast. Cleaning the Colon is vital for survival. The Colon is a part of the gut which is essentially our 2nd brain. It holds onto leftover waste and materials that create inflammation in the body and directly trigger many symptoms of disease. Without a clean colon, the body cannot function well as a whole.

Ginger Tea: Ginger is consumed in large dosages during this example of a liquid fast as Ginger is known for reducing feelings of nausea, sickness, stomachaches, muscle soreness, and strengthening the digestive system. Ginger tea is a safe option that contains many benefits while liquid fasting. You may experience many of the symptoms mentioned above in which Ginger can help reduce the severity as you push through your comfort zone to complete this 5-Day liquid fast.

Blood Cleanser Tea: 2-3 pieces of Sarsaparilla (dried herb), 1 tablespoon of Burdock, and 1-2 pieces of Guaco (dried herb). This tea supplies the body with an adequate amount of Iron which helps to filter out toxins that are in the blood. When the blood is deficient in Iron, this allows for toxins that are consumed to be spilled over into the bloodstream when the liver and kidneys are not able to filter waste materials out of the system. This tea you can drink at any time, but it is best to consume at the halfway point or closer to the end of this 5-Day Liquid Fast to allow your body to adjust to consuming liquids so it can prepare for absorbing necessary nutrients it needs to enhance the removal of toxins from the body. Consuming this tea towards the end of this fasting example, will help you feel more energized during a time that you would begin to feel more fatigued. There is no place in the body where blood does not flow. It is vital to keep the blood clean. When the blood is clean, the body can function better and be able to detect any potential issues that may be present much faster. If there is a condition that may be an underlying issue for your body, detecting it quicker by keeping the blood clean allows you to address these concerns much earlier.

Lung Support Tea: 1 teaspoon of Elderberry, 1 Tablespoon of Mullein, 1 teaspoon of Dandelion Root, 1 piece of Palo Guaco, and ½ teaspoon of Wild Cherry Bark. These herbs help clear out mucus in the lungs and helps prevent coughing, colds, chills, migraines, and joint pain. Removing mucus from the lungs and proving relief for the lungs will help enhance the experience of remaining mindful of your breath while fasting. Breathing easier will also prevent feelings of dizziness during your fast. Ending your liquid fast by improving your breathing even more will boost your confidence and help you begin working towards breaking your fast and sticking to your plan that you have set for yourself.

Water: Spring Water only. Tap water and most name brand waters contain unnatural chemicals and materials that do not help the body. There is no such thing as "new" water on our planet. Water on Earth replenishes itself through evaporation, condensation, precipitation, and collection (also referred to as The 4 Stages of the Water Cycle). Natural spring water is best and most pure for the body. Our bodies are mostly water (roughly 60%) whereas certain organs are composed of over 70-80% water. The water our bodies are made of, do not have a need for chemicals or unnecessary materials. We need to consume clean water so the water in our bodies remain clean.

Soups

Something that is not often used as often during a Liquid Fast are, Soups! Making a soup and consuming the broth (or mixing into a liquid) is a great way to use different ingredients that satisfy your taste buds as you stick to your liquid fast. All fasting methods or routines should be enjoyable. If you are not enjoying yourself, this is a sign to end your fast and revisit what may work for you. A liquid fast can be very demanding especially to a beginner. Soups can help bridge the gap between only drinking liquids, to also being able to develop some normalcy with using utensils while consuming something. Another great thing about making a soup (and consuming a whole food, plant-based diet) is that if you do not cook anything enough, the foods are often MORE beneficial for you! Raw plants have an abundant amount of benefits and can help you adjust to making things such as soups without the fear of anything being undercooked and leading to any serious health concerns.

Homemade Chickpea Soup

Ingredients:

3 cups of cooked chickpeas blended with 2 cups of spring water.
½ cup of Watercress
2 yellow peppers (chopped)
1 big red onion (cut up and sauté in grapeseed oil)

How To Make:

1. Take 3 cups of cooked chickpeas and blend with 2 cups of spring water,
2. Sauté chopped yellow peppers, ½ cup of water cress, and 1 onion together.
3. Start boiling 6 cups of spring water in a separate pan.
4. Put sautéed vegetables into pot of boiling water with the following herbs and spices (1 tablespoon of cayenne pepper and achiote, 2 tablespoons of sea salt, ½ teaspoon of thyme, 1 teaspoon of basil, ½ teaspoon of sage, ½ teaspoon of oregano and 3 tablespoons of onion powder.
5. Mix together and add blended chickpeas.
6. Let simmer for 1 hour
7. Let cool and enjoy.

Vegetable Broth Soup

Ingredients:

½ cup of Okra
1 chopped red onion
1 full butternut squash (chopped into cubes)
1 ¼ cup of turnip bulbs
add 3 cups of Spring Water (add more if needed)

How To Make:

Cook ingredients until boil, then simmer for 1-hour, stirring ingredients every 10 minutes.

Add seasonings 5-7 minutes before completing the cooking time.

Seasonings are: ½ teaspoon of Sea salt, 1 teaspoon of dried basil, ½ teaspoon of dried oregano, and add thyme and cayenne pepper to taste.

Either strain out items or blend together before adding to a bowl for soup.

Roasted Butternut Squash Soup

Ingredients:

1 full Butternut Squash cut into small pieces (halved vertically and remove seeds)

¾ cup of chopped onion

Scallions (or other leafy green vegetable)

Seasonings: Dry Basil, Dry Oregano, Thyme, Sea Salt, Ground Ginger, Achiote (powder)

How To Make:

1. Cut 1 Full Butternut Squash into cubes and season with dry basil, oregano, Thyme, sea salt, ground ginger, Achiote, and roast in the oven for 30 minutes.
2. After roasting add to a pot with water add ¾ cup of chopped onion and small handful of scallions or other leafy green vegetable (chopped).
3. Bring to a boil and taste to see if salt or spices is to your taste or if you need more.
4. Boil on low heat until it thickens then purée with a blender. Garnish with fresh herbs you enjoy.

"Gazpacho" Soup

Ingredients:

4 Roma Tomatoes
1 Cucumber
½ Green Bell Pepper
¼ Cup of Cilantro
¼ Cup of Red Onions (chopped)
½ teaspoon Cayenne Pepper
1 teaspoon Onion Powder
2 teaspoons of Key Lime Juice
¼ teaspoon Dry Basil
¼ teaspoon Dry Oregano

*Add Sea Salt to taste

How To Make:

Add all ingredients into blender. Blend until it is a smooth texture. Let sit in fridge for at least an hour before consuming.

Alkaline French Onion Soup

Ingredients:

2 tablespoons of Avocado oil
3 larger white or yellow onions (cut into half-moons)
3 larger Thyme Sprigs (about 1 tablespoon), leaves stripped (about ½ teaspoon)
2 tablespoons of key lime juice (or you can use 1 tablespoon of tamarind paste)
4 cups of recommended vegetable stock (no added salt)
2 cups of spring water
3 teaspoons of sea salt
½ teaspoon of powdered pepper
1 Bay Leaf

How To make:

1. Heat 1 tablespoon of avocado oil over medium heat into a large pot.
2. Add chopped onions, thyme leaves, 1 teaspoon of sea salt, and drizzle the remaining 1 tablespoon of avocado oil over the onions.
3. Low heat to medium/low (onion will cook down in size if they appear too large for the pot).
4. Cook without a cover, stir occasionally until onions caramelize and turn light golden brown (about 50-60min total).
5. Add 2 tablespoons of key lime juice and cook until it is absorbed (about 15min total).

6. Add the vegetable stock, bay leaf, remaining sea salt and pepper, then bring to a boil.
7. Turn the heat on low and simmer for at least 30min.
8. Remove bay leaf before serving.
9. Enjoy!

30 Day Full Body Herbal Detox

(Follow this 30 Day protocol while fasting from solid foods for optimum results. You may use any of these methods to approach difficulty in areas identified at any time Caution: make sure to gradually increase your tolerance of fasting and doing extended fasts prior to attempting this full body herbal detox from start to finish.)

Mix herbs mentioned in each section together and drink in tea form (warm or cold). Dried herbs can be mixed in a cup and have boiling water poured on them and let cool off together. Powdered herbs can be mixed well together and be added to warm or cold water, added to a juice or smoothie, or put together in capsule form.

Days 1-7 (Digestive System)
Cascara Sagrada (dried: 1tsp; powder: 1/2tsp)
Rhubarb Root (dried: 1tsp; powder: 1tsp)

Wormwood (dried: ½ tsp; powder: 1/2tsp)

Drink: Tamarind Juice.
Boil Tamarind Pods and pull out the strings and outer shells. Place inner Tamarind fruit into boiling water. Remove seeds after cooled off. Blend together and enjoy!

Drink: Papaya Smoothie
Wash and remove seeds from Papaya fruit. Cut into small pieces, blend together, and enjoy!

Follow this protocol daily for digestion relief.

Days 8-14 (Blood, Liver, and Kidney Function)
Yellow Dock (dried: 2-4tsp; powder: 2-3tsp)
Chapparal (dried: 1/2tsp; powder: 1/2tsp)
Nettle (dried: 1tsp; powder: 1/2tsp)
Elderberries (dried: 2-3tbsp; powder: 3-4tsp)

Detoxifying organs will begin to expel harmful toxins from the body while cleaning out waste materials in the body.

Days 15-21 (Rid The Body of Calcification)
Nettle (dried: 1tsp; powder: 1/2tsp)
Elderberries (dried: 2-3tbsp; powder: 3-4tsp)
Red Clover (dried: 1-2tsp: powder: 1tsp)

Body will work to expel excess mucus and reach into its' reserves for nourishment, helping the body maintain homeostasis when fasting.

<u>Days 22-30 (Replenish Minerals)</u>
Sea Moss (as much as you like)
Bladderwrack (dried: 1tsp; powder: 2tsp)
Nettle (dried: 1tsp; powder 1/2tsp)
Blessed Thistle (1/2tsp: powder 1/2tsp)
Blue Vervain (dried: 1tbsp; powder: 3tsp)
Guinea Hen Weed (dried: 1tsp; powder: 1/2tsp)

The body will work to absorb necessary minerals it needs for optimal function while also replenishing the cells that may have lost minerals during this fasting/detoxing period.

By the end of this 30 Herbal Detox You Will:

- Cleanse the intestines and colon
- Provided Liver and Kidney Support
- Cleanse blood and nervous system
- Provide more oxygen delivery to the blood and brain
- Nourish internal organs
- Strengthen immune system
- Repair nervous system
- Remove toxins from the body

Water Fasting

Similar to Liquid Fasting, only liquids are consumed when Water Fasting. The main difference is that Water

Fasting only allows for one liquid to be consumed; Water. Water Fasts typically only last for about 2-3 days. Anything more than this can create more harm than benefits that Water Fasting provides. Water Fasting helps to promote autophagy that your body works to break down and recycle old, potentially dangerous parts of your cells. Most people drink two to three liters of water per day during a water fast.

As with any fasting method, you should refrain from eating a large meal upon completing a water fast. Breaking this fast with juices and smoothies will be best as you gradually test your tolerance of consuming semi-solid and eventually solid foods.

Preparing for a water fast includes gradually decreasing the size of your meals throughout the day over the span of a few days. As you have a new normal portion size for your average meal, you will be able to begin consuming an adequate amount of water as you transition to only consuming water. Many people will often begin doing a liquid fast as they transition to a water fast to help the body adjust to this method more easily, although these individuals should already be use to liquid fasting as this will extend the number of hours and days that you are without solid foods.

Although there are several benefits from Water Fasting, one of the main risks is that you can become dehydrated during this time period. This may sound strange, but about 30% of our water intake comes from the foods we eat. Removing foods is the equivalent of subtracting 30% of our water intake when doing a water fast. We must replace this percentage of water with consuming more water, while being mindful of how often we excrete liquids through urination to make sure we are properly hydrated.

Caution: If you have an eating disorder or have had difficulties with regularly eating, it is advised to refrain from Water Fasting as recovering from this type of fast can be more difficult and trigger symptoms of an eating disorder.

It is also not clear on how Water Fasting can interact with medications a person takes regularly. If you are on medications, it would be best to use other fasting methods and routines more frequently until you are able to work your way away from medications before attempting or building up to a Water Fast. One day of Water Fasting may not be detrimental to your health, but one day is also not going to rid your body entirely of a condition or sustain a solid habit. Healing is a process that comes in many forms. Water Fasting may help but more so in your future if you are currently on medications or have a preexisting eating disorder or condition.

Dry Fasting

Dry fasting involves not consuming any solid foods or liquids. The best way to prepare for a dry fast is to hydrate properly in the days leading up to it. The body, like most other things, requires training and preparation for this kind of fast. Having adequate experience with other fasting methods is the best form of training. Eventually working up to a full day of dry fasting, and then proceeding to do a several day or longer dry fast would be the next step(s).

You want to not have as many toxins in the body as possible when Dry Fasting. If you have toxins in your body and attempt a Dry Fast, you will almost immediately feel fatigued, have headaches, feel nauseous, and will possibly catch a cold or sickness of some sort due to how your immune system responds to this change. Whenever you are doing a fast, the body will reach for its reserves at times to maintain homeostasis (balance) within the body. While fasting, the body would typically acquire nutrients throughout the day when you do consume liquids or solid foods, and cravings may come about due to any minerals you may be deficient in. When Dry Fasting, you do not acquire the nutrients you need, and your body will only be able to reach in for its reserves for nourishment. It may take some Calcium from the bones, or some Iron from the blood. For the body to do this, you will want to have enough minerals in the body at a full capacity for the body to take things from it without it hindering the performance or daily functioning of your body. The body taking minerals from different areas of the body is often what it does whenever someone is very low in particular minerals due to an unhealthy diet that does not feed the cells or nourish the body.

Over time, the body will become malnourished which creates the foundation for disease. When Dry Fasting, having enough minerals and nourishment in your reserves will prevent any illness or sickness from occurring during your fast. As the body reaches for its reserves, it will also reach for the toxins and waste materials that you want the body to focus on identifying on identifying for their removal from the body. As this process occurs, cholesterol levels will stabilize, blood sugar levels will become normal, and things such as insulin sensitivity will increase leading to insulin being absorbed by the body which is a great benefit for those who have Diabetes.

If you are still adjusting your diet and working towards a healthier lifestyle, it is not recommended that you attempt a Dry Fast.

The preparation for a Dry Fast tends to be different than any of the other fasting methods mentioned so far. Hydrating prior to starting this type of fast is crucial. It is often recommended that you do not attempt a Dry Fast for more than 12hrs the first time to avoid your body from experiencing moderate to severe side effects such as nausea, pain, muscle soreness, or exhaustion.

Dry Fasting is often performed best when your body becomes more adapted to periods of not consuming anything. This is achieved by regularly following various fasting methods, or Dry Fasting for smaller portions of your day.

For this fasting routine, there is no calendar to review as you will not have times to consume anything liquid or solid. You should, however, have a calendar available for you to track when you began your Dry Fast so you can keep track of how many days you have fasted for. If you lose track of days while Dry Fasting, this can be very detrimental to your health. It will become hard to decipher any hunger pains or fatigue from potentially harmful health concerns.

Stick to one of the fasting methods or routines mentioned in this chapter at a time. Feel free to experiment and explore fasts you feel are the most beneficial for you at this time.

An important aspect of fasting is often testing your body and how it responds to some changes. Doing a Cleanse and/or a Detox based upon your current state of health will allow you to experience the full benefits of fasting. After building up a tolerance to fasting, you can incorporate a cleanse or detox while you are fasting, or to break your fast.

In the next several pages, we will explore the differences between Cleansing, and Detoxing, in their relationship to Fasting followed by some examples of each that you can include into your lifestyle on a more regular basis when you are not fasting.

CHAPTER 9

Cleanses and Detoxes

While fasting, we are essentially cleansing the body and allowing the detoxifying organs to fulfill their duties and responsibilities. The word "cleanse" and "detox" are often used interchangeably so we will go over their main differences as well as provide some sample cleanses and detoxes you can do when you are not fasting or are working towards building your way up to starting a fast.

A *Cleanse* is a process or period of time during which a person attempts to rid the body of substances regarded as toxic or unhealthy, typically by consuming only water or other liquids. A cleanse will kickstart the body towards getting accustomed to consuming items that work towards removing harmful substances.

Doing a cleanse can come in many forms but primarily work to help the body's digestive tract.

A *Detox* is the physiological or medicinal removal of toxic substances from a living organism, which is mainly carried out by the liver and kidneys. Additionally, it can refer to the period of withdrawal during which an organism returns to homeostasis after long-term use of an addictive substance. Doing a detox will strive to support the body's natural toxin-elimination processes.

In short, a cleanse will support the digestive tract needed to function properly to begin the elimination process, while a detox will focus on specifically removing waste and supporting its own detoxification processes through the liver, kidneys, lungs, and skin.

The goal is to always rid the body of toxins which starts with removing things that are detrimental to our health. Completing a cleanse helps initiate the removal of toxins currently in our system. However, toxins like to hide out in areas of our body as they scavenge for their own survival (which comes from continuing to consume toxins). Doing a detox will help assist the body with removing these items on a deeper level prior to fasting.

First, begin by trying some of these cleanses and detoxes that will be listed to test your body on how you may adjust to a fast by getting a more personal and adequate assessment of your overall health.

<u>Sample 3 Day Master Cleanse</u>

Ingredients:

Spring Water
2 teaspoons of Key Lime Juice
2 teaspoons of Agave Nectar
1/8 teaspoon of Cayenne Pepper Powder
8oz of Natural Spring Water

Mix all these ingredients together and drink first thing in the morning.

Also make sure to "Flush" each morning as well after drinking a Master Cleanse Drink:

Each morning add 2 tablespoons of non-oxidized sea salt to 1 quart (32oz) of room temperature water. You will have to go to the bathroom about 30-45min after drinking this. You can begin drinking this as you are leaving for work or school. You do not have to finish all 32oz of it all at once, but this should get you started for the day and closer to a daily recommended gallon of water daily.

You should use this cleanse to begin to rid the body of toxins as you transition to a whole food, plant-based diet while removing processed foods. The body has difficulty absorbing minerals from food when you have a lot of toxins in it which leads to cravings. If you are not eliminating processed foods while you are doing this cleanse, you will end up back in the same position you are now in.

TIP: make recipe and fill up a pitcher of water and then ether fill a few water bottles or a gallon jug you can take with you during the day to make this readily available to drink while at work, school, etc.

Sample 3 Day Liquid Detox

Breakfast (AM):

1 cup of Spring water
1 tablespoon of Hemp Seeds
1 Cup of Raspberries
1/2 cup of Dandelion Greens
1 Burro Banana
1 tablespoon of Tahini Butter
2 teaspoons of Key Lime Juice

Lunch:

1/2 cup of Walnut or Hemp Milk
1/2 Cucumber
1 cup of Kale
1/2 Green Apple

1 Squeezed Key Lime
1 tablespoon of Coconut Oil
1 cup of Mango

Dinner (PM):

1.5 cups of Coconut Water
1 cup of Blueberries
1/2 Cup of Mango
1 Cup of Kale
1 tablespoon of Key Lime Juice
1/2 Avocado
1/4 teaspoon of Cayenne Pepper Powder
1 tablespoon of Hemp Seeds

Notice how this 3 Day Detox is different than the 3 Day Cleanse? The cleanse can be fit into the day within your normal schedule while you make dietary adjustments. While the 3 Day Liquid Detox is working to provide relief to the digestive system by limiting the overall consumption while also providing the body with an adequate amount of nutrients and minerals with the items included in each drink. When doing a Cleanse, you can still eat as you normally do with meals you usually eat. However, when doing a Detox, you are also working to remove and/or restrain from anything that may backup the digestive system or anything that is detrimental to your health.

Cleanses

Watermelon Cleanse

Ingredient:

Watermelon (as much as you want)

Duration: 2-5 days

A watermelon cleanse involves just consuming watermelon. You can blend up watermelon (preferably seeded), juice a watermelon, or a combination of the two. You will want to consume watermelon as a liquid for hydration in addition to drinking natural spring water daily. You can use watermelon as a snack throughout the day.

Consuming an abundant amount of watermelon while limiting consumption of many solid foods will adequately hydrate the body while supporting the digestive system.

You can easily turn this cleanse into a fast by ONLY consuming watermelon by eating it, juicing it, or blending it into a smoothie over the span of 2-5 days. A watermelon fast would mean the only item you consume is watermelon. You can still drink spring water during a watermelon fast, but no other foods or liquids are allowed.

Completing this cleanse will help to remove debris within the colon, while the extra water from this fruit will pick up additional toxins and expel them from the body.

Colon Cleanse

Duration: 5-6 consecutive days at a time.

Ingredients:

Cascara Sagrada (1 teaspoon)
Black Walnut hull (1 teaspoon)
Rhubarb Root (1 teaspoon)
Prodijiosa (1 teaspoon)
Water 8oz (boiling)

*You can do any combination of these herbs or take individually for this cleanse. You do not need every ingredient, but this cleanse works best when including all herbs mentioned above.

This cleanse is probably the most important to our health. The colon is essentially our second brain and is a part of the large intestine which works to remove waste from the body. The colon is responsible for holding a temporary storage of feces, but also reabsorbing water and minerals necessary to our health.

The Colon is made up of four parts:

- Ascending colon (right colon): Works to absorb remaining water and nutrients from indigestible material.
- Transverse colon: This is the middle part of the colon. Absorbs water and electrolytes while moving waste towards descending part of the colon.
- Descending colon (left colon): Stores the remains of digested foods.
- Sigmoid colon: Hold feces until the body is ready to go to the bathroom.

If the colon is not healthy, this can lead to flatulence, going to the bathroom repeatedly, stomach pains, etc. These may not seem very scary or signify an immediate response but, these can turn into underlying difficulties leading you towards disease, can lead to mineral deficiencies as the body will not hold onto essential nutrients it needs if you are using the bathroom repeatedly, can reduce blood flow to this area of the body, leading to an accumulation of dead blood cells and harmful bacteria. Not allowing these to be removed from the body, they can make their way into the bloodstream and lead to various blood disorders, can sit around and fester leading to conditions such as fibroids, a need to have lymph nodes removed, and/or cancer spreading throughout this section of the body.

Nourishing Cleanse

Ingredients:

1/4 watermelon
2 tablespoons of sea moss gel
Fresh burdock root (1 teaspoon of powder)
Fresh ginger root (1 teaspoon of powder)
1 whole key lime
1/2 teaspoon cayenne pepper powder
Add water until mixture is about 32oz.

Blend all ingredients together, drink up, and enjoy.

This cleanse is a good option for those who have not completed a cleanse and have concerns of not getting enough minerals and adequate nutrients. Sea Moss gel contains 92 of the 102 minerals our bodies are made of, while the burdock root, ginger root, and cayenne pepper powder, provide additional nourishment of minerals to the body. The watermelon and key lime, along with spring water helps to keep you hydrated as well when consuming this smoothie.

You do want to have a few days in a row where you are drinking this smoothie. Preferably 4 days in a row will allow you to use the entire watermelon and will be sufficient enough to help cleanse the digestive system while nourishing the cells.

Mineral (Powder) Cleanse

Ingredients:

1 Cup of Bladderwrack Powder
1 Cup of Sea Moss Powder
1 tablespoon of Burdock Root Powder
Get each of these in powdered form. Mix together and store in a sealed container.

You will want to take about 3 tablespoons of this mixture and make you own capsules. For this, you should use size 000 capsules and make sure you have a capsule machine that fits size 000 capsules. Take 3 teaspoons of mixture and add to capsule machine to make you own capsules. Take between 4-6 capsules 2-3 times a day.

If you do not have a capsule machine or intend on taking capsules, you may want to do more of a juice fast or incorporate this mixture into a cleanse.

You can take 1 tablespoon of mixture and add to a fruit smoothie along with 1-2 cups of natural spring water (depending upon which fruits you use; if they are watery fruits, the one cup of water will work well).

Detoxing

Detoxes are often completed as a person has built up their tolerance to fasting or has completed a few cleanses.

Detoxing is more of a process although you will hear many people refer to doing a "Detox" as opposed to simply "Detoxing". There is not always a direct start and end time to a detox. It is a process. A Cleanse can be a one time thing, while Detoxing often lasts for 7 or more days minimum.

This process involves eating fresh fruits and vegetables, herbs, juices, smoothies, and enough water daily. Consuming these items will naturally help remove waste and allow the body's detoxifying organs to function more productively and help first, to remove toxins from the body, followed by regenerating itself, resulting in the body healing itself. You want to drastically decrease or remove items such as alcohol, liquor, junk foods, candy, carbonated drinks, meats, artificial sugars, and starches during this time. You want to provide as much relief to an already backed up, and generally unhealthy system.

There are specific herbs and ways you can help clean your detoxifying organs that you can do during this process which are included in the following pages. We will go directly to the source of how to clean each detoxifying organ (liver, kidneys, lungs, and skin) through the use of eating natural foods and using healing herbs to help you save time as you adjust to a healthier diet and lifestyle.

Your diet and lifestyle will eventually relieve congestion for these detoxifying organs and allow them to naturally do their jobs without getting backed up, clogged, overworked, or compromised by an unhealthy lifestyle. Providing support and much needed relief for these organs over time simply becomes maintenance rather than working to remove anything for an extended period of time.

If you think about it, relatively healthy people do not need to rely on a cleanse or detox to help their body function properly and more effectively. A healthy person will simply incorporate cleanses, detoxes, juices, and smoothies into their lifestyle as a part of regular maintenance. Keep in mind that regular maintenance beats damage control any day.

Next, we will go over how to support each of the detoxifying organs to properly detoxify the body:

1. Liver Support
2. Kidney Support
3. Skin Support
4. Lung Support

Liver Support

Helping to purify the Liver will directly help remove many toxins from the body, as well as shield the Liver from future damage as it works to detoxify the body. Working to promote the regular working of the Liver, will drastically reduce the chances of you being susceptible to various illness and viruses. We do, however, want to promote normal function of the Liver without any destructive synthetic substances in many commercial brand products or processed items. Therefore, the herbs mentioned in this section, will provide relief and protection for the Liver as it can help the body make progress as it cleans itself of toxins.

When the Liver is officially clean and in regular working condition, new cells along the external layer of the Liver are formed which help to purify its' health while also boosting the immune system. As this happens, you may feel a more immediate effect if you were to consume something harmful to the body that you would have not normally noticed. This is what regeneration feels like. The body naturally heals itself, so having a primary detoxifying organ in stable working condition, it will signal the body immediately when something harmful or not wanted has entered your system. Think about getting an updated security system placed in your home after relying only on security lights for years. You see those lights come on at night and are aware that something is outside such as an animal or an intruder. Other times it is just the wind blowing hard or some leaves blowing by. Your attention begins to diminish because you notice the lights go off frequently with no immediate harm.

Now, adding security cameras you can notice exactly what is outside without remaining unsure if it is an intruder, animal, or something else. These security cameras will also be able to decipher the difference between an intruder and some leaves passing by and will alert you only if there is an immediate threat. This is how the Liver will now function (again) after you have worked to clean and repair it back to its normal working condition.

Liver Detox Tea

Ingredients: Burdock Root, Sarsaparilla, and Yellow Dock. About 750mg/each (about ¼ teaspoon each herb in powder form per 8oz water). Dosage changes for dried herb to about twice this amount at least.

Burdock Root helps promote urinary tract health and healthy liver function. Promotes clear, healthy skin.

Sarsaparilla contains biochemicals called saponins that promote clear, healthy skin.

Yellow Dock is classified as a bitter herb that helps promote digestion. High in iron.

Think of a drain being unclogged and how water or leftover waste will immediately go down the drain. This detox will provide this benefit for the body. The Liver is the most basic stomach related organ that naturally detoxifies the body regularly. The Liver detoxifying the body is within the typical working function of our bodies.

Poisons often enter our bodies through our consumption of processed foods, carbonated drinks, alcohol and liquor, candies, and so forth. These items weight down the Liver and provide an additional workload to its schedule. When the Liver is overworked, it can neglect to detoxify any or all of these substances which is mostly the case when these poisons are consumed regularly.

The Liver, which is the second largest organ for our body, and has the special ability to recover itself from these lethal substances which cause damage to other parts of the body. The Liver is very resilient. However, anything can break down and lead to complications if neglected and not taken care of properly.

Kidney Support

The Kidneys are two small organs located below the ribs on either side of the spine. The Kidneys main function in the body is to get rid of excess waste, balance electrolytes we need for energy, and create hormones we need for our body to receive messages via intracellular communication.

The Kidneys most importantly need hydration at the most basic level. If the Kidneys are not hydrated regularly through eating fresh fruits and vegetables, juices, smoothies, and having an adequate amount of water flowing through it, this will slow down the production of the Kidney's operating system and can lead to the kidneys getting clogged up.

For the kidneys, herbal teas will be your best option for consuming the following herbs as you want to accompany these herbs with an adequate amount of water to keep the kidneys hydrated. Drink any of these teas separately for best results.

1. Stinging Nettle (1 teaspoon of dried herb, ½ teaspoon powder per 8oz water)
2. Hydrangea Root (tea 4-8 oz cup 2-3 times daily)
3. Palo Azul (Kidneywood) (tea 8oz no more than two glasses a day)
4. *Sambong Tea

Sambong tea preparation:

- gather fresh Sambong leaves, cut in small pieces
- wash with fresh water
- boil a 1/2 cup of Sambong leaves to a liter of water

- let it seep for 10 minutes
- remove from heat
- drink while warm 4 glasses a day for best results.
- helps with fluid retention, great for kidneys.

Sample Two-Day Kidney Flush:

This will not flush them out entirely. You can have many health complications if you flush your kidneys entirely as you will lose many things vital to your health. You want to keep the kidneys hydrated while you filter out the toxins within the body. You can do this routine somewhat regularly to promote clean kidney health while limiting other snacks and items that are detrimental to our health during this time.

Day 1:

Breakfast: Fruit Juice consisting of, 1/2 cup of berries, 2 key limes (juiced), 2 teaspoons of fresh ginger, 1 cup of watermelon, and 1 cup of Kale.

Lunch: Smoothie of 1 cup walnut or hemp milk, 1/2 cup of brazil nuts, 1/2 cup dandelion leaves, 1/4 cup berries, 1/2 apple, and 1 tablespoon hemp seeds

Dinner: Large mixed-greens salad with 1/2 cup of garbanzo beans, topped with 1/2 cup grapes and 1/4 cup of Brazil Nuts or Walnuts

Day 2:

Breakfast: Smoothie of 1 cup walnut milk, 1 frozen banana, 1/2 cup kale, 1/2 cup blueberries, and 2 teaspoons of sea moss and bladderwrack power

Lunch: 2 cups of quinoa rice topped with 1 cup fresh fruit and 2 tablespoons hemp or sesame seeds

Dinner: Large mixed-greens salad, w/ 1/2 cup garbanzo beans, topped with 1/2 cup cooked parsley and a drizzle of fresh key lime juice plus 4 ounces each unsweetened cherry juice and orange juice

<u>Skin Support</u>

The Skin is the body's largest detoxifying organ. After the Liver and Kidneys have filtered out the majority of the possible toxins in the body, the skin will either allow the remaining toxins to come through its pours via perspiration (sweating), or will be blocked as it works its way out and lead to things such as pimples, bumps, sores, cankers, rashes, fungus, and skin blemishes. When the skin looks unhealthy, it is a direct reflection of how the inside of a person's body looks. Many people will drink soda and artificial fruit juices that, although water is the number one ingredient because it is a liquid, these items do not provide adequate hydration. The body is given the task of filtering out the toxins before it can even absorb any amount of water that is provided from these items. This extra work often leads to fatigue which is why most of these drinks contain a large amount of sugars. All this does is create other issues without addressing the primary issue of hydrating the body. These substances that do not hydrate the body often causes a person to overindulge by drinking more to properly hydrate themselves. Drinking natural spring water and consuming water from fresh fruits and vegetables is how to properly hydrate our bodies. There are no shortcuts to this.

For the skin to readily display issues, this is a sign that the blood has become toxic. When the Liver and Kidneys (and other organs) are backed up from removing toxins and processing waste, much of these materials will spill over into the bloodstream. As the amount of toxins continue to build up over time, the blood becomes more toxic and this leads to numerous health conditions, where the skin signifies that a blood or skin disease or illness is present.

Let us start with examining the materials that we put onto our skin. Items such as makeup, hand sanitizer, deodorant, and lotions and creams, to name a few. All these items contain chemicals that are foreign to the body and forcefully trap in the many chemicals and toxins we should want to be expelled from our bodies.

Acne is simply a symptom of poor kidney filtration.

Dry skin is often Iodine deficiency. Dry, or flaky skin often increases as an effect of cold, dry air, especially during the winter. Low Iodine often triggers this side effect.

Thyroid hormones, which contain iodine, help your skin cells regenerate. When thyroid hormone levels are low, this regeneration does not occur as often, leading to dry, flaky skin.

Also, thyroid hormones help the body to regulate sweat. People with lower thyroid hormone levels, such as those with an iodine deficiency, tend to sweat less than those who have thyroid hormone levels within a more normal range. Since sweat keeps our skin moist, the lack of sweat might also contribute to what is causing dry, flaky skin. A study published in the *Hippokratia Medical Journal*, found that 77-percent of people with low thyroid hormone levels will experience dry skin. Same info applies with those who have high iodine. You want to get your iodine from natural sources that are found within a whole-food, plant-based lifestyle.

The Skin is the largest organ you have. It is best to treat and take care of this organ as a whole. You do not want to simply apply some face masks and consider the skin on your face to determine if your entire body is relatively healthy. You want to take care of this organ from head to toe. Your face may show clear skin, but you can have dark spots, dry skin, or rough skin on other areas of your body.

Outside of living a healthier lifestyle and consuming foods that are not detrimental to our health, there are things you can do to take care of your skin. Dry Brushing, natural Face Masks, using non-harmful deodorant, remaining hydrated, and keeping the blood clean are a few things we will go over next.

What Is Dry Brushing?

Dry Brushing is a full body massage involving a dry, stiff-bristled brush. Dry Brushing has been said to help clear up dry, flaky skin, increase circulation, and help digestion. The action of regular dry brushing is great for physical and mental clarity, and for exfoliating the skin. Dry Brushing helps to aide detoxification by increasing blood circulation and promoting lymph flow/drainage. This is especially important while fasting as it will help reduce inflammation and strengthen your connective tissues in the body, which is particularly important to be mindful of when fasting.

Dry Brushing will also unclog pores in the exfoliating process.

How To Dry Brush:

- Stand upright in your bathtub.

- Start dry brushing your feet in brisk motions and make your way up, dry brushing the fronts and backs of your legs, lower abdomen, mid-section, chest, back, arms and shoulders.
- Continue dry brushing in the manner described above for about 10 to 20 minutes.
- Take a warm bath after dry brushing.
- After your warm bath, rinse yourself under a (brief) cool shower.

Anti-Acne Face Mask

Ingredients:

- 1 Key Lime (juiced)
- 1 teaspoon of Agave Nectar
- 7-10 Fresh Basil Leaves

Instructions:

- Mash fresh Basil leaves. Mix with key lime and agave nectar until smooth.
- Apply this mixture to clean skin. Allow to dry for 30 minutes. Rinse with water and pat dry.
- Repeat three times weekly.

Smoothing Face Mask

Ingredients:

- 1 Cucumber, seeded
- 1 Key lime

Instructions:

- Peel and chop one cucumber. Put the pieces in a blender and mix until smooth.
- Mix 1 teaspoon of fresh Key Lime juice with 1 teaspoon of fresh cucumber juice.
- Use a cotton ball to apply to clean skin. Leave on for 20 minutes. Rinse with cool water and pat dry.
- Repeat daily. You can store cucumber juice in the refrigerator for repeated use.

Remove Dark Spots Mask

Ingredients:

- 1 Papaya
- 1/2 teaspoon of Key Lime Juice

Instructions:

- Blend or mash up a soft ripe Papaya into a puree. Make sure there are no lumps. Add 1/2 teaspoon of Key Lime Juice and mix together.

- Apply the face mask onto your clean face and let it dry for 15-30 minutes.
- Wash away with water. You can do this as needed but no more than three times a week.

Natural Face Mask

Ingredients:

- 1 tablespoon of Agave
- 1 tablespoon of Plum Tomato

Instructions:

- Blend Plum Tomato until you get a smooth puree.
- Stir in with Agave.
- Apply mixture onto your face and let sit for about 15 minutes.
- Wash off with cold water and pat face to dry.
- For more firm skin, mix in 1 tablespoon of Sea Moss Powder and 1 tablespoon of Bladderwrack powder of this mix and leave on your face for 30 minutes before washing off.

Sea Moss Facial Scrub

Ingredients:

- 2 tablespoons of Sea Moss Gel
- Spring Water
- dry brush or exfoliating brush (optional)

Instructions:

- Add 2 tablespoons of Sea Moss Gel to a bowl.
- Add water slowly to bowl (about 1/2 cup). You can add more water if needed, but depends on preference.
- Mix together well.
- Apply Gel to face and rub into your skin. you can apply with a dry brush or exfoliating brush if you want a deeper clean.
- Wash off your face with water and pat to dry.

For this facial scrub you want to use this to clear off any dry or flaky skin, while providing the skin with some much-needed minerals to help hydrate and cleanse this area. The skin on the face is important to take care of since it is thinner than the skin in most other areas of our bodies. We want to be firm with the skin on the face, but not too rough. The face being clean helps to keep out toxins and dirt from being absorbed into the body. Our eye brows and eye lashes help to keep dirt and other materials out of our eyes, but often, these materials make their way into the skin on our face, so it is important to keep the skin in this area clean more regularly.

Deodorant

Deodorant is something the average person will use daily, especially those who are active or when it is during some of the warmer months. However, many commercialized brands of deodorant contain many chemicals and ingredients that we do not want in our body. Our skin absorbs what we put onto it. Placing chemicals harmful materials will not help our health. Common ingredients that are used in most deodorants are:

- Aluminum - linked to breast cancer in women, prostate cancer for men, and Alzheimer's disease.
- Propylene Glycol - can cause damage to the central nervous system and heart. This is a byproduct of fossil fuel found in Anti-Freeze.
- Triclosan - Classified as a pesticide by the FDA (Food and Drug Administration). Has been banned in soaps but can be used in other products.
- Phthalates - Linked to higher risk of birth defects and disrupts hormone receptors.
- Butylated Hydroxytoluene (BHT) - May cause damage to the liver, kidneys, and lung tissues.

- Parabens - May lead to early puberty in children, increase breast cancer risks, and decrease sperm levels in males.

As you can see, there are several harmful chemicals placed in deodorants. You may find a deodorant that does not contain these chemicals but has several others that are harmful to the body that have yet to have much research on them. Just like our lifestyles, we want to simplify and remove anything that may be detrimental to our health.

Natural Deodorant (Option #1)

Ingredients:

- 1 Key Lime (cut in half)
- 1-2 teaspoons of Coconut Oil

Instructions:

- Rub key lime on your underarms and pat to remove liquid from running down.
- Massage in with a small amount of coconut oil. If you feel a slight burning sensation when you apply your key limes, wash off with water and use less next time.

Natural Deodorant (Option #2)

Ingredients:

- ½ cup of Coconut Oil
- 1 tablespoon of Sea Moss Gel
- ½ cup of Shea Butter
- 1 tablespoon of Key Lime Juice

Instructions:

- Mix all ingredients together and store in a glass airtight container overnight.
- Mix well together before each use.
- Use 1 teaspoon of mixture and massage in and pat to dry.

These natural deodorants are simple and easy to use for all ages. These deodorants will not clog up our sweat glands as many deodorants do. When we sweat, our body is filtering out toxins and materials that it needs to detoxify. Trapping these materials in regularly as our sweat increases (warmer weather, exercise), this will create an increased likelihood that there will be skin issues or deterioration. When we eat correctly our bodies will naturally have a better system set in place to support the detoxifying organs so they can work effectively. Using processed deodorants filled with chemicals, will only add to the workload of our detoxifying organs. Think about completing several tasks during your workday, only to have someone give you several other tasks to do every time you complete a task. Our organs cannot pass these additional tasks off to anyone else and be forced to do this themselves, which often leads to them being backed up and overworked which can result in them breaking down and losing their effectiveness of processing and detoxifying items that can be detrimental to our health.

While fasting, our body will be removing some toxins more regularly through the skin as the rest of the body is limiting its' daily function. If you are active while fasting, or feel you will have a busy day, go ahead and try out these forms of natural deodorants to further promote your health and longevity by not holding onto or trapping toxins that should be expelled from the body.

Staying Hydrated

The most essential parts of maintaining healthy skin is by reducing and eliminating toxins from being absorbed into the body, and staying/remaining adequately hydrated. Drinking an adequate amount of water is necessary throughout our daily lives. However, something that is often overlooked, is the amount of water that we absorb through the foods we consume. Eating fresh fruits and vegetables enables our bodies to become accustomed to holding onto the water we consume. You may notice at first, that when you first begin setting a goal to drink more water, you will end up urinating more often. As your body becomes accustomed to this, it will work to hold onto the water you consume from what you eat and drink so that your body remains hydrated (you will also not urinate as much as when you are used to drinking more water daily).

While fasting, you will learn the importance of remaining hydrated as well as an important lesson: To drink your foods (juices, smoothies), and to eat your water (fruits and vegetables). As you incorporate this lesson into your lifestyle more often, you will notice that your body remains hydrated while being properly nourished, and fasting becomes a normal part of your lifestyle. Nourishing the body will feed the cells enough so that you are naturally not hungry at times and end up fasting by default.

Keeping The Blood Clean

If your blood is clean, your skin will be clean. Many toxins in the body are often pushed into the bloodstream, which is on display when we notice acne, blemishes, have dry, flaky skin, or notice marks on our skin. After initially removing these toxins from your lifestyle, you want to keep the blood clean and purified. There is not a single section of the body that blood does not flow to. Keeping the blood clear of toxins, while feeding it the Iron that it needs, is essential to its' health. What is necessary to understand with the blood is that the blood is iron. Iron is the lifeforce that supports the blood flow throughout the body. However, we must consume Iron-Phosphate which comes from plants, not Iron-Oxide which comes from heavy metals and are present in items such as artificial supplements, processed foods, and prescription pills.

Foods High In Iron:

Quinoa
Wild Rice (not black rice)
Chickpeas
Kale
Nuts (particularly Walnuts)
Hemp Seeds
Dates (and Date Sugar)
Dried Apricots
Watercress

Herbs High In Iron:

Sarsaparilla (highest concentration of Iron than any other plant)
Burdock (or Burdock Root)
Guaco
Chickweed

Fasting is a great time to work in many of these herbs as well as directly experience the many benefits these herbs provide the body.

Lung Support

Your lungs are pink, spongy organs. Inside each of them there are tubes, called bronchi, that branch out into smaller and smaller tubes. These tubes must get really small because all together you have about 1,500 miles of airway tubing! At the very end of the tubes are tiny sacs called alveoli. You have about 300 million of these.

In the tiny air sacs is where the chemical exchange, oxygen for carbon dioxide, takes place. The air sacs give up their oxygen into the blood stream, which at about the same time, gives up its carbon dioxide to the air sacs. The blood was a dark color when it arrived, but now it is leaving bright red again, thanks to its new supply of oxygen. The blood carries the oxygen on its way, and now the lungs have a new job, to send the carbon dioxide up to your nose to be exhaled.

A dome shaped muscle just below your lungs, called the diaphragm, makes your lungs breathe in and out. When your diaphragm pulls down, it leaves space for your lungs to expand, and air pressure brings more air in. When your diaphragm relaxes, the space gets smaller and air is pushed out.

The lungs' function is to convert inhaled carbon dioxide into oxygen and give this to red blood cells and circulated throughout the body. The oxygen from the inhaled air passes into the blood via alveoli. Then the CO_2 (carbon-dioxide) is taken to other parts of the lungs where the air is exhaled. Each of the two lungs have protective membranes called "pleura" that cover the lungs. When we breathe air in, our lungs pump the air down the air pipe (trachea) which splits evenly into the left and right lungs. The two tubes which transport the air into the lungs split in half a total of 22 times (bronchi) which produces more than 10,000 smaller tubes (bronchioles). These bronchioles then lead to more than 300 million air sacks (alveoli).

The trachea starts at the back of the mouth and branches to form two bronchi. One bronchus goes into each lung. Each bronchus branches many times getting smaller and smaller to form tubes called "bronchioles". All these tubes have cartilage rings for support, except the microscopic ones. At the end of the bronchioles, are the "alveoli". Each alveoli is folded on top for a set of interconnected spaces. There are many alveoli, providing an exceptionally long surface area for gas exchange. The alveoli are surrounded by blood capillaries transporting blood to and from the lungs. Cleansing the lungs improves the body's ability to connect and function each bodily system with one another.

Lung Support Tea

Ingredients:

Mullein
Dandelion Root

Elderberry
Palo Guaco
Wild Cherry Bark

You can drink these herbs together or separately. Mixing these herbs together should be done with caution as you will want to use a small amount of each herb (about ½ tablespoon per 8oz.)

Mullein herb is used to treat coughs, tuberculosis, bronchitis, hoarseness, pneumonia, earaches, colds, chills, flu, fevers, allergies, tonsillitis, and a sore throat. Other uses include, treating asthma, diarrhea, colic, gastrointestinal bleeding, migraines, joint pain, and gout.

Dandelion Root helps boost the immune system's response to upper respiratory illnesses and disorders impacting the lungs. Can reduce symptoms of asthma, bronchitis, wheezing, and respiratory infections.

Elderberry also helps to boost the immune system, ease viral respiratory symptoms, and works to break down mucus in the bronchial tubes.

Palo Guaco cleanses the bronchial tubes and is a natural cough suppressant employed for all types of upper respiratory problems including, bronchitis, pleurisy, colds, flu, coughs, and asthma, as well as for sore throats and laryngitis.

Wild Cherry Bark is used for treating lung issues, digestion relief, and is often used in syrups because of its sedative, expectorant, and cough-suppressing effects.

If you like to play competitive sports, dance, swim, or just keep active, you will want to keep your respiratory system in top shape, starting with its' main function, the lungs. Being able to breathe in lots of oxygen and holding onto carbon-dioxide makes it easier to do any activity. What you need to breathe in big breaths of oxygen is a strong and healthy respiratory system. The two primary things that are good for your lungs and the rest of your respiratory system are (1) exercise and (2) not putting anything into your lungs that is bad for them.

Aerobic exercises make your lungs strong and make you breathe in more oxygen. In fact, the word "aerobic" has to do with your muscles using oxygen. Of course, you do not have to set a timer and do 1/2 hour of jumping jacks or other aerobic exercises every day. Any activity that gets you moving are good. Just getting outside is a good start. Most people seem to think of more active things to do once they are out in the sunshine, and away from the TV and other electronics.

Some things are just not good for your lungs. These include things that you are allergic to, pollution, and cigarette smoke. Anytime you inhale smoke, it goes directly into your lungs to then have the carbon-dioxide filtered out. Why give your lungs this extra task to complete? Smoking is unnecessary and is harmful for the lungs to be able to allow your body to breathe.

Inhaling smoke can severely damage your lungs. Cigarette smoke in particular, kills many thousands of people every year. Smoking weakens the lungs' ability to function well and causes 87% of the lung cancer in the United States. It causes other diseases like emphysema and bronchitis. It increases your risk of having a stroke, a heart attack, and mouth cancer. Lung and other respiratory system damage are caused by chemicals that are in all forms of smoke (yes, this includes smoking Marijuana, even cooking foods on most pots and pans). Your Trachea is lined with little hairs, called "cilia", which filters the air you breathe to keep dirt out of your lungs. Chemicals in the air when smoke is present damage the cilia so they cannot work as well. Inside your lungs are many tiny air sacs that manage the job of getting oxygen from the air to the rest of your body. All forms of smoke break down the walls of these air sacs. After smoke has damaged lots of cells in a person's lungs, cancer cells may start to grow instead of more good cells.

Lots of smokers try to quit. Some are successful, but many are not. Some people quit for a while, but then begin smoking again. Beating the habit is not easy, because addiction to smoking affects a person both physically and mentally. According to the American Cancer Society, 90% of new smokers are children and teens. This is especially sad because we already know how hard it is to stop smoking. So, if you do start cleansing your lungs, you are doing yourself a wonderful favor! With good, strong lungs to supply you with plenty of oxygen, you can take up a new habit, maybe participating in more aerobic exercises, dancing, playing a sport, or going for a daily walk, jog, or run.

Air pollution is hard on your lungs too. When there is air pollution in the area where you live, you cannot just stay away from it. There are several sources of air pollution. How lungs are impacted depends on the amount of time exposed to the pollutant, one's general health condition and activity level at the time of exposure, and the pollutant. You want to make it a priority to consume a whole-food/plant-based diet regimen due to the fact that you will be feeding oxygen-rich and carbon-rich foods to your body system/vessel.

The Importance of An Oxygen-Rich Environment

Depriving a single cell of 35% of its oxygen for 48-hours will create what is referred to as "abnormal cell growth" as it attempts to duplicate itself for its' survival. Abnormal cell growth is a phrase to describe what we come to know as "Cancer". If oxygen is not present within the body and within the cells, the body will use sugar and waste products as a food source, which causes "Cell Mutation" and eventually "Coagulation", which is when a liquid such as blood changes from a liquid to a semi-solid state. This sets the foundation for many blood issues and conditions.

Most diets consist of foods exceptionally low in oxygen (meat/animal flesh, junk foods with artificial ingredients, sugary drinks, etc). Water contains 2 Hydrogen atoms and 1 Oxygen atom per cell. Not getting enough water, low consumption of oxygen-rich foods (such as fruit and vegetables), and destructive habits such as smoking and/or living a sedentary lifestyle, is going to set the foundation for dis-ease and illness. If your vessel (body) is an oxygen-deprived environment, you become more susceptible to various illnesses and dis-eases. Having an oxygen-rich environment/vessel, allows your body to function better and maintain its structure and longevity.

Common Dis-eases related to low oxygen levels:

- Anemia
- Asthma
- Congenital Heart Defects
- ARDS (Acute Respiratory Distress Syndrome)
- COPD (Chronic Obstructive Pulmonary Disease)
- Pneumonia

- Sleep Apnea
- Lung Diseases (Pulmonary Embolism, Fibrosis).

Summary of What Happens When We Breathe:

- Oxygen goes from our nose and/or mouth down the Trachea
- The Trachea splits in half, into two Bronchi, to bring oxygen to each lung.
- Then the oxygen reaches the Alveoli.
- Each Alveoli gives oxygen to red blood cells in the bloodstream.
- Oxygen worked with the circulatory system to travel through our bodies to reach every individual cell.

<u>Etymology of Breathing:</u>

Etymology reference for the word Spirit is "breathe".

Etymology reference for the work Soul is "mind".

Etymology reference for Ghost is "Pneuma" (the lungs). (ex. "Holy Ghost = breathing through the lungs).

For the body to properly function and promote its longevity, breathing effectively is necessary. This is a great supporter of being capable of manifesting many goals or accomplishments.

The opposite of inhalation is exhalation. Our breathing

system is referred to as Respiration. To in-spire, you must breath IN. Allowing yourself to do so by cleaning the lungs will help to create the foundation for optimum health and working towards your goals. It starts with your breathing. Space is a vacuum. Therefore, for any sound/frequency to be produced, there needs to be air so that this air can collapse on itself in the form of sound or vibration. With little to no air present in the body, how can your words make it somewhere so that it becomes audible for another recipient to cast a response back into your direction? Speak LIFE back into your body and your cells by allowing it to absorb and use its organs to maintain a high frequency.

Your body is a temple just like the mind is its own temple. Improving the function of your lungs and your ability to breath allows you to inspire yourself in ways that you understand yourself, thus, increasing the rate at which you are inspired. An individual who is frequently inspired will continue to grow and will transcend ordinary hindrances and limitations.

Incorporating breathwork into your lifestyle and deep breathing exercises is also important for supporting the lungs. In the next chapter there are some examples of breathwork and breathing exercises you can include into your lifestyle.

CHAPTER 10

Breathe

Breathing is our rhythmic pattern connecting our physical bodies to the universe. We breathe without much conscious effort. However, the way we breathe and understanding how we MUST breathe are two different things. Most people breathe through their mouths and sparingly through their nose. This can create many problems. In this chapter we will examine how breathing through our nose is the correct and most beneficial way we must breathe for our health and longevity. While fasting, it is crucial to breathe properly to help the body maintain its positive rhythmic pattern as you strengthen your connection to the universe.

25-50% of the world's population are "mouth-breathers" according to James Nestor, author of

Breathe: A New Science Of A Lost Art. James identifies in his book that "mouth breathers" are more prone to developing serious life changing issues. "Mouth breathers" are more likely to develop issues impacting the neurological and respiratory systems. Issues such as snoring, sleep apnea, adenoid face (is a condition in children who primarily breathe through their mouths where they develop a "long face"), speech issues, and many more. Breathing through the mouth can also change the structure of a person's jawline and facial structure.

Doctors of Speech Language Pathology at Stanford University conducted a study for those who got a Laryngectomy (holes drilled in the throat for a person to breathe), found that those who had this procedure, their noses were essentially closed up and blocked so they could not use it anymore for breathing. Within 2 years and 2 months their nasal passages were completely blocked. Just like any other muscle, if you do not use it, you lose it. The tissues in their noses began to close and surround the nostrils, blocking air from going in, leading to habitual mouth-breathing.

Breathing only through the nose not only sends more oxygen to the brain, breathing through the nose helps to open the CO_2 pathways and humidifies air in the body.

CO_2 (carbon-dioxide) has gotten a bad rap as we mostly hear about it when getting news about air pollution, global warming, or a poisonous substance. However, CO_2 is necessary for our survival, particularly when we breathe.

Depending on how we breathe, we are working to store CO_2 within our bodies, not just fill up our lungs with oxygen. We can do both of these things when breathing through our noses daily. When we breathe through our mouths, we are off-loading CO_2 in the body, which decreases the circulation and oxygen absorption in the body. Just filling up your lungs does not mean your body is holding onto the oxygen or that you are breathing correctly. Olympic coaches have often had runners hold a certain amount of water in their mouths as they run to help train their bodies to breathe through their nose to help improve their endurance and cardiovascular health.

You need a positive balance of oxygen and CO_2. That professional athlete you see on the sidelines breathing in oxygen from a machine is only supporting their belief that breathing in oxygen will replenish their body and help them get their breath back. This could not be further from the truth! This oxygen they are breathing in does not have anywhere to go without CO_2. Using some form of oxygen machine, will reduce how much CO_2 that is available, especially when fatigued. These athletes will not absorb much of the oxygen they are breathing in which will lead to them getting fatigued soon after re-entering a game and either become very dependent on these machines for brief periods of time, or they will suffer from cramps or other oxygen-deprivation conditions. These machines, although having good intentions, are more of a placebo than anything else; unless an athlete is guided to focus on inhaling through their noses. These athletes would be better off sitting down, drinking water, and breathing long, deep breaths through the nose. These machines function similar to social Oxygen Bars or bottles of oxygen being sold around the world as they provide less contaminated oxygen, but without CO_2, oxygen has no place to go to be absorbed within the body.

The nasal passage is the size of a billiard ball, or small fist. There is a lot of space to breathe through the nose. You can actually breathe less, and fill the body with oxygen. Breathing through the nose also produces nitric oxide, which helps battle of viruses and pathogens. You can eat right and exercise regularly throughout your life, but if you do not breathe correctly, you are drastically decreasing the health in the body.

You cannot directly control how your organs operate, but you can influence their functions through breathing.

Indian Yoga and Meditation guru Swami Rama grew up doing yoga and meditation from the age of four. On command he could make his heartbeat 300 times a minute and get his heart rate back to normalcy through his breath. *Tumo* is a common breathing practice used to build heat in the body especially in cold temperatures. Several Monasteries going back 1,000-1,200 years would use this technique to stay warm and work towards enlightenment mentally and physically. Swami Rama himself has been reported to be able to change the temperature of each finger on the same hand through breathing practices!

Today, in Boulder, Colorado there is a university (Naroba University) which is a Buddhist-inspired and mindfulness focused university which practices and studies the *Tumo* breathing practice.

Dr. Herbert Benson is an American medical doctor, cardiologist, and founder of the Mind/Body Medical Institute at Massachusetts General Hospital (MGH) in Boston, MA. He is a professor of mind/body medicine at Harvard Medical School. At Harvard, Dr. Benson and his team of researchers tested monks in the 1980s and confirmed that through breathing, one can control their heart rate and the warmth of their bodies. Monks were also able to slow down their metabolism while warming their bodies. There are videos where someone has a wet towel thrown on them and they can dry off the towel within a short time period because they are so warm, even while wearing very minimal clothing. Monks that were studied described visualizing a fire in their belly, breathing in and out, picturing the fire expanding as their breaths got deeper to warm their bodies.

Located in the Indus Valley of North India (dating back 4,000-5,000 years) there are statues doing yoga poses with their stomachs out signifying breathing exercises. This is one of the many ways researchers date many of these breathing methods that are in writing today. This society had no political or religious buildings and were considered to be an undeveloped society for their lack of social-economic development. Although, with research being revisited, it appears they held value in things that we have chosen to neglect in modern times which has created many problems that did not exist in their culture.

We seem to view hunger-gatherer societies such as those in the Indus Valley as less than because they do not have the many things we consider to be luxuries in our current lifestyles. They had to search, hunt, grow their own foods, and relocate on command due to weather or famine. However, hunters and gathers would often spend about 3-4 hours a day putting together meals and generally have the rest of the day with no distractions. Some would work on improving their hunting methods to save time, while others would seek to limit their physical activity by resting. This is how many mindfulness activities became a staple in many cultures as they would want to limit physical activity while repairing the body. Breathwork came into more direct practice as they had to prepare for long expeditions, fasting, not wasting energy, and working to remain quiet while hunting animals.

When you hold your breath and feel a need to breathe, this is not due to oxygen; this is CO_2 (carbon dioxide) decreasing. Having this understanding helps to show how Magicians are able to remain calm when doing underwater tricks and have to hold their breath for an extended amount of time.

When you see a horse running full speed or a cheetah hunting down its prey; they are not breathing from their mouths. Your dog or cat cools their body down through breathing through their nose via thermo-regulation. Animals have an entire system in their bodies to help unconsciously cool themselves down but, we humans have the conscious ability to do the very same activity.

Breathing through the nose provides a higher threshold of CO_2. It sends signals to the amygdala (area of the brain) which dictates fear. When breathing through the nose, you become more comfortable with fear and can remain calm without panic. This remains particularly helpful in hunter-gatherer societies and high-level activity such as Mixed-Martial Arts, or mountain-climbing.

The idea the people should breathe more when

they panic is exactly the opposite. Take for instance someone who experiences panic attacks, anxiety, or has asthma. During these experiences, they begin to hyperventilate, in an attempt to secure and hold onto more oxygen. What they do not realize is that, when you increase the speed of your breath, you are off-loading CO_2 which your body needs to hold onto oxygen. Off-loading CO_2 causes more constriction and makes it more difficult to breath, often leading to someone losing consciousness and passing out. Anyone who feels and attack coming on, slow breathing through the nostrils is needed. Sending oxygen straight to the brain (specifically the amygdala which controls fear), while not off-loading CO_2 will allow a person to remain calm as their body processes this experience, and fully recover while retaining their consciousness.

Being triggered to hyperventilate due to overstimulating events is a condition that is an inflammatory response. The body tries to respond to a stimulus, but is unable to process it, leading to a triggered response that involves low CO_2 retention and oxygen absorption and hyperventilation. The brain struggling to process a series of events is due to inflammation in the brain.

Many foods that are consumed today did not exist a few decades ago. These processed and inflammatory producing foods limit oxygen absorption in the brain as well as impairs the respiratory system and the breath in the body which influences mouth breathing. Foods that require more chewing, or chewing much throughout the day can influence how our jaws are shaped and influence how we breath. Think about how many times you chew as well as the quality of the foods you eat (snack foods) and how these foods impact your teeth. Foods detrimental to our health (junk foods) negatively impact our teeth, which also influence our jaw shapes and how we breathe. Chewing these foods throughout our life span can also lead to developing a thicker neck and thicker tongue due to inflammation, making people more prone to developing sleep apnea, sleep paralysis, and sleep with their mouths open. Eating healthy foods (often easier to chew) that protect our teeth, in turn, protect our jaw shapes, will allow us to breathe through our nostrils much easier as we work on making this adjustment.

If you find yourself having many meals each day or being persuaded by food cravings, this is due to mineral deficiencies. Eating foods high in mineral content, you can eat less while providing your body proper nourishment and make fasting a more regular part of your daily life. This also highlights the importance of consuming foods that contain oxygen in the form of H_2O.

Dr. Justin Feinstein (Clinical Neuropsychologist at the

center of Laureate Institute of Brain Research) and his team are currently studying CO_2 and its connection to conditions such as Anxiety and Asthma. Dr. Feinstein and his team have conducted studies to address how these conditions (anxiety, asthma, and stress) can be reduced by taking a shot of CO_2 to offset the stress receptors that trigger the symptoms of these conditions rather than practicing breathing techniques to have a more immediate effect. Anyone who experiences Anxiety, Asthma, or internal stress, have shown to have an extreme low threshold of CO_2. So, by taking a shot of CO_2, Dr. Feinstein wants to close the gap as well as the time span in which people can recover and reduce these experiences. Similar techniques appear to be beneficial for those with allergies as well.

At Stanford University, studies on nostril breathing have been proven to be more beneficial than mouth breathing. Cyclists that were tested who would normally breathe 47 breaths per minute were able to breathe 14 times per minute which increased their endurance, performance, and recovery. According to Zara Patel, MD, a Rhinologist and Otolaryngologist at Stanford Medicine, the lungs cannot utilize the air breathed in through the mouth as effectively, because it is not warmed or humidified as it is when you breathe through your nose.

The *Wim Hof Method* developed by a man named Wim

Hof ("The Iceman") has gained popularity recently as this method is based on the belief that you can accomplish incredible feats by developing command over your body through use of specific breathing techniques.

Wim Hof himself has achieved incredible feats such as, climbing some of the highest mountains in the world while wearing shorts, standing in a container while immersed in ice cubes for nearly two hours, and swimming below ice for 57.5 meters (188 feet, 6 inches). Hof ran an entire marathon in the Namib Desert without drinking water and ran a half marathon north of the Arctic Circle with bare feet.

Hof has the belief that anyone can accomplish similar feats through controlling their breathing which allows for more self-control, better blood circulation, and improvements regarding inflammation, anxiety, stress, sleep quality, and boosting the immune system. Following the *Wim Hof Method*, there has been studies such as a group of twenty-six trekkers who climbed Mt. Kilimanjaro found that the Wim Hof Method helped to reduce Acute Mountain Sickness (AMS) while also reversing some of the symptoms of AMS as they appeared. Scientific research is continuing to increase in the field of breathwork due to individuals such as Wim Hof.

In Wim Hof's online platforms and app, participants learn a variety of breathing techniques, yoga, meditation, and can participate in ice baths (if applicable). Applying these techniques daily, all contribute to improving the quality of your breath.

A woman referred to as the "Peace Pilgrim" (Mildred Lisette Norman) walked more than 25,000 miles over the span of twenty-eight years in her efforts to increase peace on Earth. She would walk often at heights above 18,000ft and for more than nineteen hours or longer without food or water. Mindfulness and breathing techniques were a primary focus for her expeditions. In her book, *Steps Toward Inner Peace*, she mentions how important purifying the body is for her expeditions and how much of her purification came from long periods of time embarking on an expedition with no food or water. Through focusing on the breath and not relying on much or any foods (fasting), the Peace Pilgrim was able to set forth on pushing through extensive mental and physical barriers.

She was quoted in her texts as stating, "As long as you work for your selfish little self, you're just one cell against all those other cells, and you're way out of harmony. But as soon as you begin working for the good of the whole, you find yourself in harmony with all your fellow human beings. You see, it's the easy, harmonious way to live".

Let us now work though some breathing exercises

you can make a part of your daily routine starting on the next page.

Breathing Exercises:

(Some of these are adapted from James Nestor's Book *Breathe: A New Science Of A Lost Art*)

30 Nostril Breathes

For this exercise, you will simply take a total of 30 breaths by breathing in and out only using the nostrils 30 times. Focus on increasing how deep your breath gets during this exercise to avoid feeling light-headed or dizzy.

If you do begin feeling light-headed or dizzy at any time, you may stop this exercise and hydrate by drinking water to help recover.

If you need a visual aid feel free to look at each number as you inhale and exhale until you are completed with this exercise

1 2 3 4 5 6 7 8 9 10 11 12 13 14 15 16 17 18 19 20 21 22 23 24 25 26 27 28 29 30

Pursed Lip Breathing

This simple breathing technique makes you slow down your pace of breathing by having you apply deliberate effort in each breath. You can practice pursed lip breathing at any time.

How To Do This Exercise:

- Relax your neck and shoulders.
- Keeping your mouth closed, inhale slowly through your nose for 2 counts.
- Pucker or purse your lips as though you were going to whistle.
- Exhale slowly by blowing air through your pursed lips for a count of 4.
- Repeat until satisfied.

Alternate Nostril Breathing

Alternate nostril breathing is a yogic breath control practice. In Sanskrit, it is known as *nadi shodhana pranayama*. This translates as "subtle energy clearing breathing technique."

This exercise works to lower stress, symptoms of anxiety, increase CO_2 (Carbon-Dioxide) absorption within the body, and can improve cardiovascular health.

You can practice alternate nostril breathing on your own, but you may want to ask a yoga teacher to show you the practice in person so you can make sure you're doing it correctly.

Focus on keeping your breath slow, smooth, and continuous to help you to remember where you are in the cycle.

How To Do This Exercise:

- Sit in a comfortable position with your legs crossed.
- Place your left hand on your left knee.
- Lift your right hand up toward your nose.
- Exhale completely and then use your right thumb to close your right nostril.
- Inhale through your left nostril and then close the left nostril with your fingers.
- Open the right nostril and exhale through this side.
- Inhale through the right nostril and then close this nostril.
- Open the left nostril and exhale through the left side.
- This is one cycle.
- Continue for up to 5 minutes.
- Always complete the practice by finishing with an exhale on the left side.

Diaphragmatic Breathing

Belly breathing can help you use your diaphragm properly. Do belly breathing exercises when you are feeling relaxed and rested. Practice diaphragmatic breathing for 5 to 10 minutes 3 to 4 times per day. When you begin you may feel tired, but over time the technique should become easier and should feel more natural.

How To Do This Exercise:

- Lie on your back with your knees slightly bent and your head on a pillow. You may place a pillow under your knees for support.
- Place one hand on your upper chest and one hand below your rib cage, allowing you to feel the movement of your diaphragm.
- Slowly inhale through your nose, feeling your stomach pressing into your hand. Keep your other hand as still as possible.
- Exhale using pursed lips as you tighten your stomach muscles, keeping your upper hand completely still. You can place a book on your abdomen to make the exercise more difficult. Once you learn how to do belly breathing lying down you can increase the difficulty by trying it while sitting in a chair. You can then practice the technique while performing your daily activities.

Breath Focus Technique

This deep breathing technique uses imagery or focus words and phrases. You can choose a focus word that makes you smile, feel relaxed, or that is simply neutral to think about. Examples include peace, let go, or relax, but it can be any word that suits you to focus on and repeat through your practice. As you build up your breath focus practice you can start with a 10-minute session. Gradually increase the duration until your sessions are at least 20 minutes.

How To Do This Exercise:

- Sit or lie down in a comfortable place. Bring your awareness to your breaths without trying to change how you are breathing. Alternate between normal and deep breaths a few times. Notice any differences between normal breathing and deep breathing. Notice how your abdomen expands with deep inhalations. Note how shallow breathing feels compared to deep breathing. Practice your deep breathing for a few minutes.
- Place one hand below your belly button, keeping your belly relaxed, and notice how it rises with each inhale and falls with each exhale.
- Let out a loud sigh with each exhale.
- Begin the practice of breath focus by combining this deep breathing with imagery and a focus word or phrase that will support relaxation. You can imagine that the air you inhale brings waves of peace and calm throughout your body. Mentally say, "Inhaling peace and calm." Imagine that the air you exhale washes away tension and anxiety. You can say to yourself, "Exhaling tension and anxiety."

4-7-8 Breath

The 4-7-8 breathing technique, also known as "relaxing

breath," involves breathing in for 4 seconds, holding the breath for 7 seconds, and exhaling for 8 seconds.

This breathing pattern aims to reduce anxiety or help people get to sleep. The 4-7-8 breathing technique requires a person to focus on taking a long, deep breath in and out. Rhythmic breathing is a core part of many meditation and yoga practices as it promotes relaxation. Dr. Andrew Weil teaches the 4-7-8 breathing technique, which he believes can help with the following:

Reducing Anxiety
Helping a person get to sleep
Managing Cravings
Controlling or reducing anger responses

Dr. Weil is a celebrity doctor and the founder and director of the University of Arizona Center for Integrative Medicine.

How To Do This Exercise:

- Before starting the breathing pattern, adopt a comfortable sitting position.
- To use the 4-7-8 technique, focus on the following breathing pattern: empty the lungs of air
- Breathe in quietly through the nose for 4 seconds
- Hold the breath for a count of 7 seconds

- Exhale forcefully through the mouth, pursing the lips and making a "whoosh" sound, for 8 seconds
- Repeat the cycle up to 4 times

Lion's Breath

Lion's breath is an energizing yoga breathing practice that is said to relieve tension in your chest and face. It is also known in yoga as Lion's Pose or simhasana in Sanskrit.

How To Do This Exercise:

- Come into a comfortable seated position. You can sit back on your heels or cross your legs.
- Press your palms against your knees with your fingers spread wide. Inhale deeply through your nose and open your eyes wide. At the same time, open your mouth wide and stick out your tongue, bringing the tip down toward your chin.
- Contract the muscles at the front of your throat as you exhale out through your mouth by making a long "ha" sound. You can turn your gaze to look at the space between your eyebrows or the tip of your nose.
- Do this breath 2 to 3 times in a row a few times.

Resonant or Coherent Heart Breathing

Resonant breathing, also known as Coherent Heart Breathing, is when you breathe at a rate of about 5 full breaths per minute. You can achieve this rate by inhaling and exhaling for a count of 5. Breathing at this rate maximizes your heart rate variability (HRV), reduces stress, and, according to one 2017 study, can reduce symptoms of depression when combined with Iyengar yoga.

How To Do This Exercise:

- Inhale for a count of 5.
- Exhale for a count of 5.
- Continue this breathing pattern for at least a few minutes.

CHAPTER 11

Why Your Powers Increase When Fasting

Every ancient healer has taught that food regularly in the alimentary tract interferes with our natural connection with the chemical elements of Cosmic Radiation. Food in the body insulates the body against the natural contact of Cosmic Radiation by corroding the poles of the cells. That obstruction causes the function of the body cells to decline below the higher level of functioning.

As this damaging condition of insulation is increased by regular eating, the vital force of the body gradually decreases, and decrepitude slowly appears.

Then comes that time in due course when the function of the cells within the body decline more and falls below the life level of vibration, resulting in the condition called "death". What must be better understood is that illness and disease are symptoms of death. This explains the secret and little-known reason why man's health and all his powers increase and grow more acute under a fast. Limiting intake, limits symptoms, and reduces risk for disease and illness.

During a fast, the alimentary tract becomes free of the insulating effect of food, and the cells can free themselves of the damaging corrosion.

This permits the body to make more and better use of the chemical elements of Cosmic Radiation, produces an increase in cell vibration, and puts the condition of the body back nearer to the normal state in which it was before man fell to the level of the animal plane by forming the habit of eating off of impulse and availability.

Fasting permits the body to clean house, purify its fluids, normalize its chemistry, and regain its proper equilibrium. This is regeneration.

The body cannot regenerate itself when it is full of inflammation, mucus, parasites, toxic metals, and excessive hormones provided by consuming items that are detrimental to our health.

When fasting, you become more aware and in tune with how habitual the act of eating has become. Many of us do not eat for hunger, we eat for pleasure. The absence of constant pleasure exposes you to emotions that you mask with your habits, and you are finally exposed to who you really are. Now the healing process can begin. Physical, emotional, and spiritual transformation is now within your grasp.

The late healer Dr. Sebi (Honduran Herbalist and Healer), Robert Morse (Physician, Biochemist, and Herbalist), Arnold Ehret (German Naturopath best known for his Mucusless Diet Healing System), Hippocrates (Greek Physician), all the way back to Imhotep (Ancient Egyptian Physician, Architect, and Astrologer) all have reported that the purer the body, the less it craves food. When the body is perfectly free of toxins and in normal working condition, the need for food practically vanishes. This allows the body to repair and replenish the cells of what they need. The body can take a more accurate assessment of what it needs and be able to better prepare itself for rejuvenation and protecting itself from viruses and potential illness.

Notable Checkpoints To Do Daily:

- Check the urine at regular intervals to see if the kidneys are filtering.

- Drink plenty of water to help flush the system, however if you notice that urination isn't occurring, despite drinking lots of water, then have some dandelion, hawthorn or horsetail herbal tea; these are diuretics and can be used in instances where the body is holding on to fluids.
- Cleansing the colon is important; always start with this first.
- Practice deep breathing exercises daily.
- Do not use things on the skin you would not eat or drink.
- Do not drink water straight from the tap, filter your water.
- Do not shower with regular, store bought soaps as these will only further irritate the skin
- Understand that you must work to keep the body healthy.
- Adopting a whole food, plant-based diet going forward will help you to maintain general health and wellness. Even before the end of a fasting period one should begin to see positive results

CHAPTER 12

Final Thoughts

Fasting will do things for you that cannot be explained through verbal language. You will feel emotions leave your body as you develop a newfound connection with what you consume and the emotions you give. As you release these, you will feel lighter and happier. Your temperament will feel more balanced and you will know when and how to re-connect with the foods you choose to consume.

You would be amazed how much the body opens up and the energy levels you reach the deeper you get into your fast, it is truly amazing.

Every time you have a bowel movement while fasting, you begin to cleanse, heal, detox, and repair each system with the body. Your channels of elimination, the bowels, liver, kidneys, and skin are key in unlocking the body while healing. Healing is not overnight; it is a process just like anything else so trust it.

Set your mind to it and focus. Nothing should be able to break you from your goals if you want it enough. Only you can stop yourself. Strive for perfection and always set your own standards.

When you look beyond religion this customary practice of fasting is not only good for our spirit but also highly beneficial for health and longevity.

Fasting is an innate human behavior. For our ancestors, three square meals a day was not always guaranteed. There was often one large meal eaten when food was available, and the circumstances were safe. Is it possible that we are more suited to these ancient eating habits than our usual routine of breakfast, lunch, and dinner?

Fasting may seem like a tough thing to do, but we all fast every day (well every time we sleep). Also remember that the word breakfast literally means to "break" or end a daily fast. Healing is not an overnight process. It is a daily cleansing of pain. It is a daily healing of your life.

We must use fasting as a tool in helping us reach longevity and optimum health. We must work to make diseases a thing of the past. We must eat foods the way that nature has made them so that we can remain the way that we were made; not deteriorate and become unrecognizable due to illness and disease.

Our consumption of toxins does not match our elimination rate. This is why many suffer from disease and illness. What comes in does not always leave. It stays in the body and festers because the digestive system is backed up. We must first change the ratio of toxins coming in and the rate of toxins coming out as we all work towards a healthier lifestyle which promotes quality and longevity. All of this is to be thoroughly promoted by the ancient practice known as, *Fasting*.

REFERENCES

Adams, Mike. *Food forensics: The hidden toxins lurking in your food and how you can avoid them for lifelong health*. BenBella Books, Inc., 2016.

Al Tameemi, Wafaa et al. "Hypoxia-Modified Cancer Cell Metabolism." *Frontiers in cell and developmental biology* vol. 7 4. 29 Jan. 2019, doi:10.3389/fcell.2019.00004

Ayoub, Noel, et al. "Nasal Symptoms Following Laryngectomy: A Cross-Sectional Analysis." *American Journal of Rhinology & Allergy*, vol. 34, no. 3, 21 Jan. 2020, pp. 388-393, 10.1177/1945892420901631. Accessed 6 Oct. 2020

Berger, Ralph J., and Nathan H. Phillips. "Energy conservation and sleep." *Behavioural brain research* 69.1-2 (1995): 65-73.

Cahill Jr, George F. "Ketosis." *Kidney international* 20.3 (1981): 416-425.

Cotes, John E., David J. Chinn, and Martin R. Miller. *Lung function: physiology, measurement and application in medicine*. John Wiley & Sons, 2009.

Coutinho, Luke, and Sheikh Abdul Aziz Nuaimi. *The Dry Fasting Miracle: From Deprive to Thrive*. Penguin Random House India Private Limited, 2020.

Dasgupta, Ananya, et al. "Intermittent fasting promotes prolonged associative interactions during synaptic tagging/capture by altering the metaplastic properties of the CA1 hippocampal neurons." *Neurobiology of learning and memory* 154 (2018): 70-77.

Dawson, Drew, and Nicola Encel. "Melatonin and sleep in humans." *Journal of pineal research* 15.1 (1993): 1-12.

Dictionary, Oxford English. "Oxford english dictionary." *Simpson, JA & Weiner, ESC* (1989).

Ehret, Arnold. Rational Fasting: For Physical, Mental, and Spiritual Rejuvenation. Book Publishing Company. 2012

Exton, J. H. "Gluconeogenesis." *Metabolism* 21.10 (1972): 945-990.

Halberg, Nils, et al. "Effect of intermittent fasting and refeeding on insulin action in healthy men." *Journal of applied physiology* (2005).

Harper, Douglas. "Online etymology dictionary." (2001): 2011.

Hof, Wim, and Koen de Jong. *The Way of the Iceman: How the Wim Hof Method Creates Radiant, Longterm Health--using the Science and Secrets of Breath Control, Cold-training and Commitment.* Dragon Door Publications, Incorporated, 2017.

Hunninghake, Gary W., et al. "Inflammatory and immune processes in the human lung in health and disease: evaluation by bronchoalveolar lavage." *The American journal of pathology* 97.1 (1979): 149.

Hurrell, Richard F. "Preventing iron deficiency through food fortification." *Nutrition Reviews* 55.6 (1997): 210-222.

Irving, M. H., and B. Catchpole. "ABC of colorectal diseases. Anatomy and physiology of the colon, rectum, and anus." *BMJ: British Medical Journal* 304.6834 (1992): 1106.

Kieffer, Dorothy A., Roy J. Martin, and Sean H. Adams. "Impact of dietary fibers on nutrient management and detoxification organs: gut, liver, and kidneys." *Advances in Nutrition* 7.6 (2016): 1111-1121.

Kong, F., and R. P. Singh. "Disintegration of solid foods in human stomach." *Journal of food science* 73.5 (2008): R67-R80.

Lockett, E.(n.d.). *Doing a natural kidney cleanse at home*. Healthline. https://www.healthline.com/health/kidney-cleanse#sample-cleanse

Lu, Zhigang, et al. "Fasting selectively blocks development of acute lymphoblastic leukemia via leptin-receptor upregulation." *Nature medicine* 23.1 (2017): 79.

Marx, Jean L. "Oxygen free radicals linked to many diseases; the oxygen free radicals, although made as by-products of normal oxygen-using reactions, nevertheless have a wide potential for causing cell injury." *Science* 235 (1987): 529-532.

Muhammad, Elijah. *How to Eat to Live*. Vol. 1. Elijah Muhammad Books, 2008.

Murray, Robert P., et al. "Menthol cigarettes and health risks in Lung Health Study data." *Nicotine & Tobacco Research* 9.1 (2007): 101-107.

Nestor, James. "Breath." (2020)

O'Brien, Justin. *Running and breathing*. Yes International Publishers, 2002.

Papagiannopoulos-Vatopaidinos, Ioannis-Eleemon, Maria Papagiannopoulou, and Vassilis Sideris. "Dry Fasting Physiology: Responses to Hypovolemia and

Hypertonicity." *Complementary Medicine Research* (2020): 1-10.

Patterson, Ruth E., et al. "Intermittent fasting and human metabolic health." *Journal of the Academy of Nutrition and Dietetics* 115.8 (2015): 1203-1212.

Peace Pilgrim. *Steps toward inner peace.* Friends of Peace Pilgrim, 1996.

Perez, Laura, Regula Rapp, and Nino Künzli. "The Year of the Lung: outdoor air pollution and lung health." *Swiss medical weekly* 140 (2010): w13129.

Pyo, Jong-Ok, et al. "Essential roles of Atg5 and FADD in autophagic cell death dissection of autophagic cell death into vacuole formation and cell death." *Journal of Biological Chemistry* 280.21 (2005): 20722-20729.

Saunders, Kerrie K. *The vegan diet as chronic disease prevention: Evidence supporting the new four food groups.* Lantern Books, 2003.

Taber, Keith S., and Richard K. Coll. "Bonding." *Chemical education: Towards research-based practice.* Springer, Dordrecht, 2002. 213-234.

Trepanowski, John F., and Richard J. Bloomer. "The impact of religious fasting on human health." *Nutrition journal* 9.1 (2010): 57.

Vásquez-Moctezuma, Ismael, Enrique Méndez-Bolaina, and Dolores J. Sánchez-González. "Skin detoxification cycles." *Indian Journal of Dermatology, Venereology, and Leprology* 78.4 (2012): 414.

von Meyenfeldt, Maarten. "Cancer-associated malnutrition: an introduction." *European Journal of Oncology Nursing* 9 (2005): S35-S38.

Wei, Min, et al. "Fasting-mimicking diet and markers/risk factors for aging, diabetes, cancer, and cardiovascular disease." *Science translational medicine* 9.377 (2017): eaai8700.

Williams, Xandria. *Liver Detox Plan: The revolutionary way to cleanse and revive your body.* Random House, 2012.

Woods SW, Charney DS, Goodman WK, Heninger GR. Carbon Dioxide—Induced Anxiety: Behavioral, Physiologic, and Biochemical Effects of Carbon Dioxide in Patients With Panic Disorders and Healthy Subjects. *Arch Gen Psychiatry.* 1988;45(1):43–52. doi:10.1001/archpsyc.1988.01800250051007

Images

Gunnars, K. (n.d.) *6 popular ways to do intermittent fasting*. Healthline. https://www.healthline.com/nutrition/6-ways-to-do-intermittent-fasting#TOC_TITLE_HDR_2

Pelz, D. (2020, July 29). *How long should you fast?* Dr. Mindy Pelz | Reset your Health | Nutrition Health Coach. https://drmindypelz.com/how-long-should-you-fast/

Soul, S. (n.d.). *The breakdown of intermittent fasting*. Seva Soul. https://sevasoulhealth.com/blogs/educate-and-practice/the-breakdown-of-intermittent-fasting

Dr. Sebi Nutritional Guide
https://drsebiscellfood.com/wp-content/themes/sebi/assets/src/nutritional-guide.pdf

ABOUT THE AUTHOR

Bryan McAskill (Ed.M., B.A.) is a Herbalist, Clinical Therapist (LMHC, LSC), natural health expert, Coach, Personal Trainer, Holistic Guider and dedicated Healer from Lynn, MA.

Follow on Social Media:

Instagram:
@bryan_mcaskill
https://instagram.com/bryan_mcaskill?igshid= bgimb1wwjz15

@herbal.healing781
https://instagram.com/herbal.healing781?igshid= 19qtcgbq8li7u

Facebook:
Herbal Healing By Bryan McAskill
https://www.facebook.com/herbal.healing781/

Printed in the United States
By Bookmasters

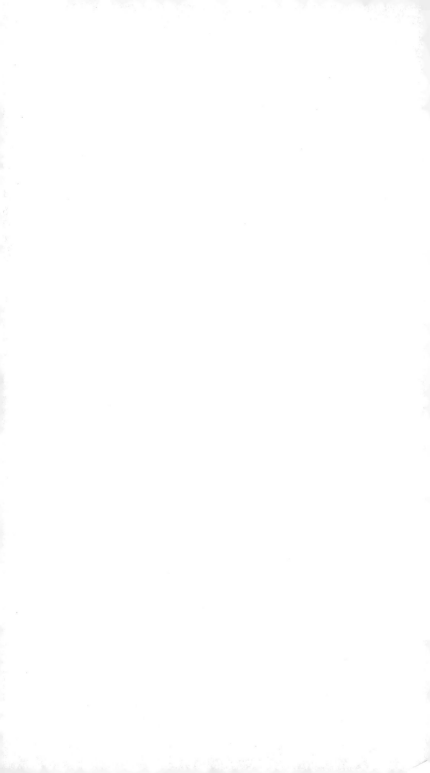